INTERMITTE.

16/

THE COMPLETE STEP-BY-STEP GUIDE TO NATURALLY LOSE WEIGHT, HEAL YOUR BODY, SUPPORT HORMONES, BURN FAT, AND LOOK YOUNGER WHILE STILL ENJOYING THE FOODS YOU LOVE.

Hannah Bailey

TABLE OF CONTENTS

Introduction 6

    What Is Intermittent Fasting? 6

    How Does Intermittent Fasting Work? 6

    The History of Intermittent Fasting 8

    Myths on Intermittent Fasting 14

Chapter 1: Why IF 16/8? 18

    What Is the 16:8 Method? 18

    The Benefits of 16:8 IF for Your Health 19

    Challenges of Intermittent Fasting 22

    Therefore, You Should 26

Chapter 2: Before Starting with IF 16/8 29

    Who Should Not Practice Intermittent Fasting? 29

    Mistakes to Avoid Committing 31

    Frequently Asked Questions 35

    The Importance of Mindset 39

Chapter 3: The Basic of IF 16/8 42

    How to Follow the 16:8 Method 42

    16/8 Method Step-by-Step 44

    What You Can Eat 46

    Foods to Avoid 50

    Managing the Macronutrients 52

    Typical Schedule for the 16/8 Method 54

    Does IF Have Different Effects on Men and Women? 61

Chapter 4: Scientific Facts About Intermittent Fasting 62

    Increased Brain Cell Production 62

    Increased BDNF Production 63

    May Protect Against Alzheimer's 64

How Intermittent Fasting Impacts Human Growth Hormone (HGH)) 64

Fasting and Leptin 66

Fasting and Inflammation? 67

Chapter 5: Exercise and Fasting 69

When to Exercise 70

Exercising Before You Eat 71

Exercising After You Eat 72

Go with What Makes You Comfortable 72

Exercising on Different Fasting Schedules 74

Chapter 6: Different Methods of IF 76

Lean-Gains Method 76

14:10 Method 76

20:4 Method 77

The Warrior Method 78

12:12 Method 78

5:2 Method 79

Eat-Stop-Eat (24-Hour) Method 80

Alternate-Day Method 81

Spontaneous Skipping Method 82

Crescendo Method 83

Chapter 7: Tips and Tricks for Staying Healthy 85

Chapter 8: Recipes 94

Breakfast 94

#1 Onion Tofu 94

#2 Spinach Rich Ballet 95

#3 Pepperoni Egg Omelet 96

#4 Nut Porridge 97

#5 Parsley Soufflé 98

#6 Bok Choy Samba.. 99

Lunch.. 100

#7 Pimiento Cheese Meatballs 100

#8 Baked Salmon with Pesto (Keto Style)............................... 102

#9 Camembert Mushrooms..103

#10 Mediterranean Stuffed Chicken 104

#11 Bacon Frittata with Kale and Potato 106

Dinner 108

#12 Western Pork Chops 108

#13 Stuffed Mushrooms 109

#14 Garlic Bread Stick 110

#15 Smothered Pork Chops 111

#16 Spicy Pork Chops 112

Snacks... 113

#17 Orange and Apricot Bites.. 113

#18 Zucchini Chips.. 114

#19 Trail Mix 115

#20 Kale Chips 116

#21 Cinnamon Cocoa Popcorn 117

Conclusion **118**

References **122**

Introduction

What Is Intermittent Fasting?

Intermittently Fasting (IF) means daily eating systems that do not consume or seriously limit calories for a longer time.

Fasting or times of voluntary food abstinence have been observed worldwide for decades. Intermittent fasting to improve relatively new fitness. Intermittent fasting means food consumption is reduced for a certain period of time and requires no changes in the food you eat. The most famous IF protocols are currently a regular speed of 16 hours and a full-day fast, one or two days a week. Intermittent fasting could be seen as a natural eating pattern that human beings have evolved into, and it traces our paleolithic ancestors. The current model of a planned intermittent fasting program can contribute to many aspects of health, from the body´s makeup to longevity and aging.

How Does Intermittent Fasting Work?

This type of fasting is not all hype with no context; there is science behind the efficacy of intermittent fasting on human health. There are many health benefits, in addition to weight loss or weight management, as discussed previously. Blood pressure, triglycerides, fat mass, blood glucose, LDL cholesterol, and blood sugars all improve as intermittent fasting becomes more and more familiar with in your body system.

Intermittent fasting has been associated with diabetes prevention and has resulted in the reprieve of pre-diabetic symptoms. Sugar is what our cells use for energy. If our cells don't use it for energy, the sugar is stored as fat within our fat cells. Sugar can only enter our cells with insulin. Insulin is what brings the sugar into our fat cells and keeps it there. Intermittent fasting lowers insulin levels, which prevents our fat cells from holding on to stored sugar in our bodies, which inevitably, if not released, causes a decrease in energy.

Like with exercise, Intermittent fasting puts your body's cells under mild stress. A physiological benefit of intermittent fasting is that your body learns to cope with this stress and fight back, hence resist disease more and more as your body learns to cope. This fasting is associated with making your bodies overall health stronger. Intermittent Fasting has reportedly been associated with an influence on metabolic regulations. This includes circadian rhythm, gut microbes, and modifiable lifestyle behaviors.

Humans have evolved to perform most physiological processes at optimal times; certain activities are optimally done during the day hours, and others, like asleep, are done at night. This is what most people call natural. A circadian rhythm is the regular recurrence of life activities in a 24-hour cycle. Consuming food outside of the normal feed phase, which is during the night hours when people should be sleep, resets some circadian rhythms and disrupts energy balance, affecting a person's metabolism. Any fasting that encourages NOT eating during the night hours, allowing the body to burn fatter synchronizes food intake with the optimal times to eat.

Having an intermittent fasting lifestyle seems to have a positive impact on gut microbiota. Gut microbiota is a complex community of microorganisms that live in your digestive tract. This positivity also goes along with the circadian rhythms. Gastric emptying and blood flow function optimally during the daytime rather than at night, so disturbing circadian may negatively affect gastrointestinal functions and ultimately impair metabolism and health.

Intermittent fasting has improved self-reported sleep satisfaction. Nighttime eating has been associated with sleep deprivation and insomnia, which can have negatively affects insulin resistance. Insulin resistance increases the risk of Diabetes and other cardiovascular diseases. The increased effects of prolonged nightly fasting can prevent Diabetes, other cardiovascular diseases, negative insulin resistance, insomnia, and sleep deprivation.

The History of Intermittent Fasting

Within the past few years, the concept of Intermittent Fasting has started to trend heavily, impacting anyone interested in dieting and healthy living. Its origins, however, are much more ancient than most of us would ever think. In this chapter, you'll be introduced to the long history of Intermittent Fasting so that you can better understand how that trajectory leads to today. By the end of this section, you should feel confident that you know where the tradition came from, as well as what it has to do with you—reading this book at this very moment.

IF for Primitive Humans

Intermittent Fasting has been a practice as long as humans have existed. In the times of our most primitive ancestors, IF wasn't so much a chosen lifestyle as it was a necessity. It came down to the prevalence and availability of food—and the hunter's and gatherer's abilities to acquire it.

In these ancient times, people would have had to go longer between meals and sometimes spend days without eating. However, what arose from necessity produced incredible and even sustainable physical, mental, and emotional effects. These ancient people would have also (likely unintentionally) been able to concentrate better, live longer, slowing age, and digest with ease consistently.

Primitive humans would also occasionally fast for shared purposes once societies and civilizations started assembling. For instance, before going off to war, communities would fast, and young people coming-of-age would fast as part of those rituals. Sometimes societies would also demand a fast as an offering to the gods or to implore the end of natural disasters such as floods or famines.

Religious Instances of IF

In the same vein as using a fast as an offering to the gods, many ancient cultures eventually required some fasting for their religious purposes. Consider Christianity. Orthodox Christians of the Greek variety still practice their ancient fasts, which comprise almost 200 days out of the year. Non-Orthodox Christians are also invited to fast whenever moved to do so to become closer to the Holy Trinity.

Consider Buddhism. The practice of intermittent fasting has always been essential to reaching enlightenment because it helps the soul undo its ropes to the body. The enlightened one, Siddhartha, practiced fasting for many years as a method o acquire wisdom.

Consider Judaism. The day before Passover, an ancient tradition followed still today that the first-born child of each family should fast to celebrate the miracle from Moses' time that spared all Hebrew first-borns. Furthermore, Jewish people are invited to fast throughout the year at any point to celebrate a life lost, to appeal to God or a prophet, or to express sorrow for a sin or wrong committed.

Consider Islam. Ramadan´s holy month features a 4-week-long fast from the time the sun rises to the time the sun sets. During this time, drinks are also shunned, as well as alcohol drinking, smoking, or performing any bad habits or repetitive practices that don't serve the soul. Muhammad, the prophet of Islam, also suggested his followers fast every Monday and Thursday, but it's unclear how consistently this suggestion is heeded.

Other religions across the world have also required a temporary fast for spiritual reasons, and it is true that many have gotten closer to their gods through this practice. However, there are so many more benefits to fasting than just these spiritual ones, and these other applications are made clear in the next chapters.

From the Past to Now

On top of being used for survival and religious purposes, intermittent fasting has gained appeal through time for its medical applications as well. Even millennia before its trending popularity today, back in 400 BC, intermittent fasting made an appearance and gained popularity by the suggestion of Hippocrates.

Yes, *that* Hippocrates! The infamous "father of modern medicine" advocated for fasting to heal almost any internal injury or state of disease. He once wrote, "To eat when you are sick, is to feed your illness," if that gives you any indication of the incredible uses he found for the practice.

Other ancient Greek philosophers, writers, and historians have echoed these concepts from Hippocrates through time into the early years, AD. Essentially, just like how animals seem to "fast" when they're getting sick or feeling unwell, humans have the same instincts but often ignore them, pushing through the illness and feeding it with food when the body needs the exact opposite.

Past the ancient Greeks, however, other thinkers across time have affirmed the same feelings. For example, Paracelsus (another founder of modern medicine) famously wrote, "Fasting is the greatest remedy," and Benjamin Franklin (one of America's founding fathers) also once inscribed in a journal, "The best of all medicines is resting and fasting."

Fasting has also been used as a form of political protest. The most famous instance of this happening occurred with Mahatma Gandhi, who lasted 21 days at his longest fasting periods. His goals were to protest against India's dependence on Britain and to acquire freedom and integrity for his people. Many others have taken up fasting for similar aims, but none have been so successful or so famous, it seems.

Contemporary Applications

Now, it seems that fasting has gained new fame in the form of Intermittent Fasting. The capital letters here are used intentionally to connote the almost "patented" application of these ancient theories about health and weight loss in recent times.

The intermittent fasting practice has been trending for the past few years, and its impact has spread widely since then. People have lost incredible amounts of weight. They've seen their energy levels improve drastically. They've been able to heal brain disorders and reverse the signs of aging. People across the world have come to understand what amazing uses fasting can have, and they are becoming healthier because of these realizations.

Doctors who have practiced fasting cures for decades have almost consistently welcomed the increased interest in IF these days, for they know how much good this practice can do for so many. Fasting is still used for religious and spiritual purposes, and some still practice it as they strive to survive. For others, IF today is revered as the so-called "fountain of youth," and many dietary plans are starting to incorporate its themes.

Overall, it seems that IF has been used throughout time for three main things: survival, spiritual connection, and body/mind health. These applications are valid today, but the focus tends toward that final point in the list: body/mind health. For those seeking a state of internal balance, IF can be a blessing. For those intrigued by IF, keep reading to find out more and to learn how to build this practice into your daily routine.

Myths on Intermittent Fasting

There are many myths out there about Intermittent Fasting. The common myths are as follows;

MYTH 1: Your body will definitely enter starvation mode.

TRUTH: Your body will not definitely enter starvation mode through Intermittent Fasting. Skipping meals or adjusting to longer periods between meals where you don't eat will not make you starve. It's going to help your body remember how to absorb nutrients. It's going to help you thrive instead.

MYTH 2: You'll lose muscle in this endeavor.

TRUTH: This myth goes along the same lines as the first one above. Just like your body won't enter starvation mode (unless something goes very, very wrong or you're trying to do too much), your body won't lose muscle through IF. The only reason why intermittent fasting would cause muscle loss would be if it were causing you to starve, but once again, the first myth addresses this falsity, making this myth false as well.

MYTH 3: You'll almost assuredly overeat during eating windows, and that's not healthy at all.

TRUTH: While some people will have the instinct to overeat during eating windows, not everyone will overeat. Even those who do at the start will realize how to move forward without this overeating instinct in the future. Your body will urge you to overeat because, in the beginning, it won't realize what you're doing to it, but as long as you keep portion sizes largely the same and don't gorge on snacks, your body will adjust, and so will your appetite.

MYTH 4: Your metabolism will slow down dangerously.

TRUTH: Your metabolism won't slow down just because you're eating less often. People who think this myth is true only assume that restricted caloric intake will make one's metabolism slow down over time; still, these individuals forget that IF isn't necessarily about cutting down calories overall. It's actually about cutting down the times during which one consumes calories. There needn't be any caloric restriction whatsoever! It just depends on the practitioner and what he or she decides to do with dieting IF.

MYTH 5: You'll only gain weight if you try skipping meals.

TRUTH: This myth is based on the same logic that drives the myth about overeating. If you gorge yourself during your eating windows, you'll surely gain weight, but hardly anyone will continuously gorge with IF. Anyone who tries will realize how unsuccessful it is, so they will not continuously gorge in response. Anyone who doesn't realize their efforts with eating is unsuccessful will soon realize that something's wrong, as their weight shows no improvement. Skipping meals never necessarily means that someone will gain weight. It just means that people who skip meals and gorge or overeat when mealtime won't see the desired effects.

MYTH 6: There's only one way to do IF that's right and truly the best.

TRUTH: This myth is absolutely and utterly false. There is no one right way to practice Intermittent Fasting, and part of the beauty of IF is that there are so many different methods, meaning each approaching IF likely has a few different options to choose from. Similarly, different body and personality types will be drawn to different methods, based on individuals' abilities and goals. IF is about flexibility, adjustment, and self-correction. There's no one right method for everyone, and there's no "best" method to strive for. Do whatever method feels right and suits your life, and once you've found it, practice it as long as you can! That's far more realistic and accessible.

MYTH 7: It's not natural to fast like that.

TRUTH: It's more natural to practice Intermittent Fasting than it is to eat three full meals each day! It's more connected to our evolutionary drives and to our primitive selves to eat like this.

And it's better for our brains, hearts, cells, and digestive systems to have a break from food once in a while to recalibrate. As you learned in the Introduction, people have been practicing Intermittent Fasting as long as humans have been in existence. It's only myths like this that circulate today that make it seem like IF is foreign, unhealthy, and dangerous. Animals of all types become healthier after periods of fasting, and humans are no different. Remember that we are animals and that IF is in our nature. Proceed with that confidence and knowledge!

Chapter 1: Why IF 16/8?

What Is the 16:8 Method?

This method, also known as the Lean-gains protocol, involves 14-16 hours of fasting with a feeding window of approximately 8 to 10 hours. This method is one of the simplest intermittent establish practices because after dinner (the last meal of the day), you go almost 16 hours fasting. During a banquet, you can easily include two or more dishes such as lunch, snacks, and dinner. For example, suppose your dinner ends before 8:30 PM. And don't have lunch until one p.m. From the next day, I already hit 16.5 hours fasting between meals! While feeding, you can eat your lunch at 1:00 PM, snacks at 5:00 PM, and then a hearty dinner at 8:30 PM and repeat the cycle.

This method can be complicated for people who are very hungry in the morning and cannot function without food. But instead of worrying about lack of food, you can consume non-nutritious drinks and lots of water to make your stomach think it´s "full," which reduces hunger.

Moreover, it is better to keep yourself busy instead of messing around or doing nothing, as this can distract your attention. One of the most important things to keep in mind is that you should avoid all kinds of prepared foods and junk foods or foods that are high in calories while eating. If you want to eat a bite or feel pain while fasting, drink two glasses of water and wait about 30 minutes. Your hunger will disappear. If you feel like eating sweets at the windows, don't look at cookies or chips or other food that is ready to eat. Instead look for something wholesome, such as carrots with yoghurt or cucumber sticks with hummus. This not only helps you to feel full but also does not add empty calories to your body! The best way to follow this intermittent fasting method is to combine it with a low-carbohydrate diet. Lack of carbohydrates helps reduce hunger and appetite and also helps to lose fat!

Just as every coin has two sides, nothing exciting or worthy can only be on one side. Despite all its advantages, intermittent fasting also has its disadvantages. Here we will see both the pros and cons of following an intermittent fasting protocol.

The Benefits of 16:8 IF for Your Health

Intermittent fasting techniques, including the 16:8 method, are most commonly used to assist in weight loss by the general population. The method has been tried by thousands of people and is also scientifically proven to be a helpful resource in reducing body fat and improving body composition. Weight loss is often considered the number one reason people opt for a diet and program that utilizes intermittent fasting.

Altering the Functioning of Body Cells and Hormones

Intermittent fasting practiced for a while brings several alterations in your body. For your body to make more fats accessible, it tends to initiate significant cell repair processes and changes the levels of hormones in your body. The levels of insulin in your body drop, facilitating the breakdown of fats. Growth hormones also increase as the blood levels in them increase a factor that facilitates muscle gaining. The body induces processes such as cellular repairing and removal of any waste materials from the cells.

Reduces the Resistance of Insulin

The common characteristics of diabetes include high levels of blood sugar in the situation of insulin battle. Thus, intermittent fasting helps in lowering the levels of insulin, which helps in preventing this illness. It also helps protect any possible damages that can affect your kidneys.

Reduction of Oxidative Constant Worry and Body Inflammation

Intermittent fasting helps reduce stress, which is one of the riskiest ways of fast aging as well as other chronic illnesses. Free radicals are the molecules responsible for reacting with molecules such as DNA and proteins and destroy them. Intermittent fasting, therefore, helps fight body inflammation and destroy any molecules responsible for constant worries.

Heart Health

Intermittent fasting is beneficial for your heart's health and prevents you against any heart diseases. Since it regulates sugar levels in your body, intermittent fasting prevents you from high blood pressure, and inflammatory markers, and cholesterol levels hence maintaining the heart health.

Induction of Cellular Restoration Procedures

When you fast, your body initiates the cell's 'waste elimination' procedures that are known as autophagy. Body cells break down and metabolize the dysfunctional proteins that accumulate inside the body cells. Increased waste elimination prevents your body against other illnesses such as Alzheimer's disease, one of the common neurodegenerative disorders with no cure.

Prevention Against Cancer

After your body eliminates any dysfunctional cells that accumulate over time, it becomes free from any cancer risks. The uncontrolled development of cells is one of the common characteristics of cancer, and therefore, intermittent fasting facilitates your body's metabolic rate, which helps reduce any possible risks of cancer. Intermittent fasting also reduces several impacts of chemiotherapy.

Brain Health

Since intermittent fasting is better for your body, then it is best for your brain. Reduction of oxidative stress and various worries is advantageous for your brain tissues. Recurrent fasting increases the development of new nerves, which improves the functioning of your brain. It also helps in increasing brain hormone levels known as the Brain-derived neurotrophic factors, which helps fight depression and any other brain-related illnesses. Intermittent fasting also helps fight brain damages caused by stroke.

Extending Lifespan

Intermittent fasting can help you live longer due to its ability to control metabolism rates, regulating blood sugar levels, and eliminating any dysfunctional cells within your body.

Challenges of Intermittent Fasting

Hunger and Food Cravings

Fasting can make hunger more intense. However, your body should get used to this side effect over time. In the beginning, you may find that food is all you think about. You may crave sugar from time to time as your body is looking for a quick energy source. It will take a bit of willpower and some of the strategies mentioned above to get past some hunger.

Your workouts at the gym may be impacted

Some people do find it difficult to perform at the same physical level on an empty stomach. If this is the case for you, it might take some additional planning on your end to avoid working out near the end of a fasting cycle. When you work out, you lose a lot of water and sodium from your body through sweat. Rehydration following exercise will be an important step in your routine.

Heartburn

Your stomach produces acid to help with digestion. Intermittent fasting impacts the production of stomach acid, which in turn can lead to heartburn. Heartburn may be worse if the eating window is later in the day. The good news is that this symptom usually goes away after a few weeks. In the meantime, it might be best to avoid eating foods that will make your heartburn worse. This includes heavily processed foods, some dairy, spicy foods, and foods that are high in acidities such as chocolate, coffee, onions, and garlic.

Headaches or dizziness

Some people experience headaches when they first begin on an intermittent fasting plan. Headaches are usually mild but may be reoccurring for the first few weeks of your transition. Dehydration will make headaches worse, so make sure you are drinking plenty of water during your fasts. You might also try adding salt to your water to make sure your electrolytes are staying in balance. See your doctor if your headaches continue for more than two weeks.

Diarrhea or constipation

The drop-in insulin levels that are associated with intermittent fasting can sometimes signal the body to get rid of excess water. The result of this may be episodes of diarrhea. In addition, eating less food may also result in less movement of the bowels. Fasting can slow down the digestive system, which may cause constipation. For both of these conditions, drinking lots of water will help. Be patient as your digestive system stabilizes and becomes accustomed to your new way of eating.

Low Energy or Brain Fog

When you first start on your intermittent fasting plan, you may feel sluggish, lethargic, or even weak at times. Keep in mind that on this plan, you are running on less fuel than you are used to. Feeling a bit low in energy is quite normal. Your energy levels may fluctuate quite a bit as you get started with the plan, but should disappear after a few weeks. You may also experience some minor difficulties in concentrating, which is sometimes referred to as "brain fog."

Hormonal Changes

Intermittent fasting affects hormone levels and functioning for women in particular.

Sleep Disturbances

Your sleep patterns and quality of sleep might be affected by this change in your lifestyle. You may find that both hunger pains and fluctuations in hormones might keep you awake at night. Your body tends to produce more adrenaline in response to a fast, as your metabolic rate receives a boost. This process may end up giving you energy at times when you would rather be sleeping or can make you feel a bit jittery.

Irritability

Changing your eating habits may affect your mood. Some people get cranky or irritable when their blood sugar levels drop. Expect some minor changes in your mood or some mood swings as you get started.

Bad Breath

A few people experience something called "keto breath" when fasting. The ketones that our body produces when in a fasted state are the cause of this nuisance. This side effect is more common for longer, extended fasts, and again, tends to go away with time.

Dehydration

Lack of eating may make you forget to take water. You might fail to take note of the thirst cues when fasting.

Fatigue

Intermittent fasting makes you feel tired, especially if you are trying it for the first time. Your body tends to run short of energy and disrupts your sleep patterns, coming along with a feeling of being tired.

Therefore, You Should

Ensure that Your Body Is Fit for Fasting

It is by making sure that you are not pregnant, not under any medication, no health complications, not underage, or even diabetic. If you cannot fast, then you can always change to cleaner eating habits such as eating natural foods and eliminate any sugar, rich, or fatty foods from your diet.

Before starting intermittent fasting, you should always consult your doctor. He will give you updates about your health concerns and advise whether the step is necessary or not.

Prepare your Household, Body, and Thoughts Before Starting Intermittent Fasting

It means that you should have enough rest and get prepared emotionally. Think about your aim and how to achieve it. Make sure that you hide or keep out of reach any food that could tempt you during your fasting period.

Stop Pretending to Be a Hero, Even When Your Body Is Weak

Do not push your body too hard in the name of fasting. There are some of the symptoms that should be of great concern during your fasting time. You should take note of heart shudders, light-headedness, and general feebleness. It requires the use of common sense because you cannot force your body to do what it cannot.

Do Not Engage in Tough Exercises; Do Light Ones

Engage in massages as they help have even blood flow in the body parts full of calories, thus reducing cortisol. Do not burn the muscles for energy while fasting.

Always Take Your Vitamins Depending on the Method of Fasting You Choose

That acts as a supplement, especially if in liquid form as it eases the process of digestion. They help compensate the vitamins lost while fasting.

Never Forget to Take a Lot of Water Every Fasting Day

Your urine should alert you if it is not light in color. If not so, drink desirable amounts of water for proper hydration.

Since you are fasting, it is an obstacle to associating with your friends who are having fun, eating chocolates, and drinking wine since you will get tempted to take some. You can indulge in other ways of having fun with your friends. You can pay a visit to the nearest mall, window-shop new clothes or electronics. Avoid grocery stores and any dinner dates. Clear any mouth-watering photos from your gallery.

Chapter 2: Before Starting with IF 16/8

Who Should Not Practice Intermittent Fasting?

Intermittent fasting is NOT recommended for people with increased nutritional needs, those with specific health problems or certain health risk factors, or those requiring substantial meals throughout the day. For example, intermittent fasting is not recommended for people:

The Very Underweight People

Excessive thinness may be a sign of difficulty absorbing the nutrients of food, and fasting would only exacerbate the situation.

The Pregnant Women and Breastfeeding

This is when they need to feed more; hence, fasting should be postponed to another period.

Adolescents and children: in the time of development, the body mustn't suffer deprivation. People who routinely take particular medications, including aspirin, metformin, or maybe blood pressure-lowering drugs, are advised not to engage in intermittent fasting.

You Are Under the Age of 18

At this age, the child is still in their growth spurt, and fasting makes nutrients necessary for growth unavailable. And this may later affect the child's cognitive and motor development. However, it will not be catastrophic if a child misses a meal or two. The most important thing for the child is to eat healthy food, not junk food, which packs the body with foreign, toxic matter.

You Have an Eating Disorder

Eating disorders like anorexia originate as a result of the fear of gaining weight. Such people tend to tightly control the amount of food they eat and exercise rigorously to keep weight off. Irrespective of how much weight they lose, anorexic maintain the fear of gaining weight. In most cases, these people are usually underweight and therefore, should not fast for their safety.

You Have Less Than 4% Body Fat

When body fat is less than 4%, you may be in starvation or malnutrition mode. In this state, it is not advisable to fast. Here's why. During the fast, your body may begin to burn proteins in the muscle tissues to keep the body alive. This will certainly weaken the body, and ultimately, you may be unable even to move. This phenomenon is called wasting and is an unhealthy condition to be in.

Mistakes to Avoid Committing

Sticking to an intermittent fasting approach will let you experience tremendous benefits, including better digestion, significant weight loss, minimal sugar cravings, better sleep, and improved mental clarity. However, your journey towards attaining your desired results will most likely be accompanied by some errors. Considered that you can't practice perfect intermittent fasting for the entire period you are planning to do it, there are some mistakes committed by other practitioners of this eating pattern that you can avoid.

Changing Your Eating Habits Drastically

If you are one of those whose regular eating habits include eating every three to four hours or so, then shrinking the time you need to eat within just 8 hours all of a sudden can lead to certain issues, like extreme hunger and frustration.

Consuming the Wrong Liquids

Some people drink tea, black coffee, or water so they can go through their fasting period with the least amount of discomfort.

If you can't tolerate black coffee, you may be tempted to add some sugar or milk without thinking about whether or not this will break your fast. Before adding anything to your drink, find out if it will affect your desired results first. If possible, do not let coconut oil and butter get near your coffee.

Start Intermittent Fasting Quickly

Many beginners make the mistake of starting intermittent fasting way too fast, and when they begin too quickly, it becomes unsustainable for them to continue with it. If you have started anything immediately, you might have noticed that it became easier for you to follow, which led you to consistency. The Same goes for intermittent fasting, and you need to make sure you take the first steps as fast as possible.

Overeat – Eat too Little During the Eating Window

People make the mistake of eating a lot or too little when following intermittent fasting, and the truth is that people who are looking to lose weight will eat less during their eating window, thinking that it will help them losing more body fat and people who are looking to gain weight will eat more thinking that it will help them gaining more weight. To be successful with I.F. you need to eat the right amount of calories and to have a balanced macronutrients intake.

Not Drinking Enough Water

Drinking water is crucial during your fasting periods. It also helps you care about your appetite. We will talk about why you should be drinking more water when intermittent fasting and show you why you might not be drinking enough water and techniques to drink more water when fasting. Many people know that water is very beneficial to humans. Water helps to detox your body clean out your system, and curb appetite. You must be drinking more water when fasting. Believe it or not, most of the time, you're drinking a lot less water than you required to be drinking.

One of the best thumb rules to follow when you are drinking water is too drink 1 oz per pound of body weight. So if you weigh 150 lbs., you should be drinking 150 ounces of water, especially when you're intermittent fasting, as water will help you forget about food.

Sticking to the Wrong Intermittent Fasting Plan or Approach

Note that for IF to produce favorable results, you need to pick the right plan that perfectly fits your lifestyle, current condition, and personality. Avoid making yourself miserable by trying to stick to a pattern, which is not compatible with your lifestyle. If you know that you are a night owl, then avoid starting your fasting sessions every 6 pm.

Beating Yourself Up in Case You Eat Beyond Your Eating Window

Do not feel too guilty if you slip up from the pattern sometimes. Avoid beating yourself up when you grab a food even if you are no longer in your eating window. Note that you need to listen to the cues sent by your body. If you feel real hunger, then there is no reason to deprive yourself of what you need.

Pushing Yourself Too Hard

This is a mistake often committed by those who wish to try extending their fast for as long as possible, even if it means forcing themselves. Some even go to the fasting extent for more than 48 hours, even if they already experience discomfort. You should determine whether the extended/prolonged fast works for you before trying it out first.

Trying to Do Numerous Things at Once

You may be forcing yourself to do many things while trying to practice the intermittent fasting approach. Some of the things you might do are over-training, dry fasting, and under-eating. Also, remember that if you are someone with poor eating habits and lacks workout in the past and want to try intermittent fasting for better health avoid biting more than what you can chew. This is important, especially if you are still a beginner.

Choosing the Wrong Foods

A lot of intermittent fasting followers also make the mistake of choosing the wrong foods. In fact, many of those who tried it think that it is a magic pill capable of solving their weight and health problems. While it is true that IF is an effective tool for those who want to have full control over their health and weight, it is still possible to cancel out its benefits if you eat the wrong foods, specifically processed and sugary ones, during your eating window.

Frequently Asked Questions

Most types of changes come with a lot of questions, and intermittent fasting is not different. Here are some frequently asked questions from beginners.

Can I have coffee?

Yes, you can have black coffee, water, and plain steeped tea.

Can I add cream/sugar/milk to my coffee?

The goal of fasting is not to add calories, so the answer is no; you should not add anything to your coffee. However, I have heard of cases in which intermittent fasters add less than 50 calories to their coffee. They have claimed to still be successful with intermittent fasting; Apparently it does not affect their fasted state, but keep in mind all individuals are not created equal. I would not recommend adding anything to your coffee, but if adding something to your coffee still makes this a good change for the goal you have for yourself, then give it a try.

Does intermittent fasting work well with veganism, paleo, keto, vegetarianism, or any other styles of eating?

Yes, the beauty of intermittent fasting is that it can be combined with any style of eating unless otherwise directed by a medical professional. You can turn your style of eating into the 16:8 method with ease, as this change does not restrict or state the style/types of food you eat. It is specifically based on the timing of your eating.

Is there an alternative to the 16:8 method if I cannot initially fast 16 hours a?

Yes, especially for women. They can start with a 14-hour fasting window and 10-hour feeding window. This is recommended for women, but men can start here if needed. Once the 14 hours is mastered, you can then work your way up to the 16:8 method.

Can I have a cheat meal?

Technically, you can eat what you want when intermittent fasting; there are no food group restrictions. There is no cheat meal to have unless you have decided that you have put yourself on some type of restrictive meals/foods to not indulge in; if so, then yes, but I recommend always eating in moderation.

What are some healthy snack foods to eat on the go during my feeding window?

- Pepperoni slices
- Fruit
- Veggie tray
- Skinny Pop Popcorn, individual bags (unless you will always measure the servings before consuming)
- Turkey/beef jerky,
- Individual peanut butter cups
- Whole-grain cereal
- Almond milk
- Eggs
- Rice cakes
- Nuts (individual bags)
- Hummus, and more.

I am too hungry during my fasting window. What should I do?

Be patient as your body adjusts to this change. This may take some time. For some, it occurs fast; for others, it may take a week or so, but this depends on how you were eating before you began this lifestyle. According to Collier, your body is still adjusting to how it was functioning before and is fighting you to get back to that way, as most people were eating more frequently and maybe even more meals or snacks during the day. Eventually, you will not feel this way. Eventually, you will adapt to your feeding and fasting windows, and the urge to eat or the thought of starving will get easier and easier until it goes away.

Why am I not losing fat faster, like other people are?

It is more than likely a combination of not eating the appropriate portions when you are eating and not preparing to eat the right food choices. Although fat and weight loss can still happen, it is more frequent and visible when the appropriate food choices and portions are selected and prepared.

How Can I Stay Full Longer?

Eat more fiber and drink more water, stay hydrated.

Do I Have to Eat Low Carb?

No, you can eat what you want during your feeding window. I recommend eating proportionately and choosing healthier food options. Instead of white bread, choose whole grain bread. Instead of white rice, choose brown rice. Instead of anything with high fructose corn syrup, scratch it off. Instead of canned fruit, eat fresh fruit.

Should I Exercise in the Fasted State?

You can, but it is not required. It is also not recommended on heavy lifting days.

What if I Am on Medications and Must Eat with My Morning Medications?

In this case, you would need to make your feeding window begin at whatever time you take your meds. I would recommend taking your meds as late as you can in the mornings but do get authorization of your plan from a medical professional.

Should I Discuss this with My Medical Professional Before Beginning the Change?

Yes, you should always discuss diet changes with a medical professional before you begin.

The Importance of Mindset

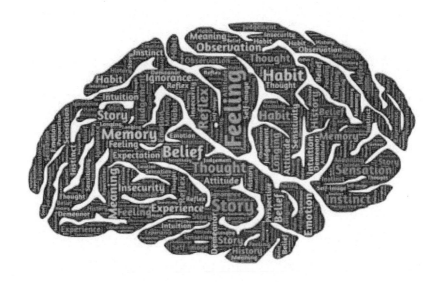

Numerous individuals don't consider the connection between a positive mindset and weight reduction achievement. Nonetheless, circumventing figuring 'I can't do this' or 'it's unimaginable for me to get in shape' will, in a roundabout way, damage your weight reduction endeavors.

A positive mindset then again pushes you the correct way every single time. On the off chance that you accept that 'I can do this' and 'I will get in shape' and afterward remain quiet about rehashing these musings, you will reliably take the activities that are essential for weight reduction achievement.

In this subchapter, I'll investigate the significance of an uplifting attitude when you need to get more fit and post the main 4 reasons why you should have an inspirational outlook while pointing toward a trimmer figure.

Your attitude likewise significantly affects your exercise execution and achievement. You'll see that you fear each exercise and won't perform at your pinnacle with a negative attitude. This will be unfavorable to your weight reduction endeavors and breaking points your general achievement after some time.

When you have an uplifting mentality, you will end up performing to your greatest potential more often than not. This will fasten your weight reduction results and permit you to accomplish your objectives in the fastest conceivable time. Furthermore, in any event, during the occasions when you don't observer prompt outcomes from your activity, you won't be disheartened as you will realize that each exercise is helping you accomplish your long haul weight reduction objectives.

On the off chance that you change your mentality to one of fun and idealism, your vitality levels will rise, and you will start to make the most of your whole weight reduction venture. You'll anticipate attempting new activities, appreciate exploring different avenues regarding new solid plans, and have a great time getting more fit.

Regardless of how much exertion you put into getting in shape, there will consistently be times when you fall off the wagon and experience mishaps. With a negative frame of mind, these mishaps can crash your weight reduction endeavors and cause you to struggle reaching your goals.

An uplifting attitude limits the effect that a difficulty has on your weight reduction venture. Rather than feeling that your weight reduction routine is never getting down to business and that you are burning through your time, you'll acknowledge every mishap as it comes, gain from it and push ahead.

Chapter 3: The Basic of IF 16/8

How to Follow the 16:8 Method

The 16:8 method is very flexible, and that means you can choose your own specific 8-hour eating window, according to your day. You might work shifts, and that means you sleep at different times. What you should do in that case is pick an 8-hour window, which is when you are mostly awake. Obviously!

For example, if you are working nights and sleeping between the hours of 10 am and 6pm, you can eat from 6 pm until 2 am. You would then probably be working until the following morning when you would head off to sleep, but you could drink coffee (unsweetened and black) to keep you going also, and plenty of water. This might not work for you, so you could think about shifting your pattern and starting it later, perhaps if you don't feel like eating the moment you open your eyes. You could then choose an eating window of 9 pm and eat freely until 5 am.

It's not only about when you can eat, but it's about what you eat too. While there are no restrictions and no lists of foods you must eat and foods you shouldn't, always remember that if you suddenly pile a huge breakfast or lunch on your plate after fasting, you're going to end up with stomach ache. That could mean that you end up eating too many calories within your eating window and put weight on, or you end up with stomach disturbances for the rest of your eating window.

So, how many calories should you eat? It depends on whether you want to lose weight or maintain. A standard calorie amount to maintain weight is 2500 calories per day for a man and 2000 calories per day for a woman. This does depend on the height, current weight, and metabolism of the person and is only an average, healthy amount. If you want more solid guidelines on your specific circumstances, speak to your doctor, who will be able to give you a calorie aim plan tailored to your needs.

Within that calorie amount, you should make sure that you get a good, varied diet. That means proteins, carbs, fats, vitamins, and minerals. Again, we're going to cover what you can and what you can't eat, loosely because there are no rules, but varied is the way to go. Ironically this will also help you enjoy your new lifestyle more because you're not bored and eating the same things all the time. This is a pitfall many people suffer from regular low-calorie diets; the change is so restrictive that they end up eating the same thing day in, day out, and over time they get so bored and rebel against it. This usually ends in a binge day, which causes extreme guilt and then leads them to throw the diet in the bin and go back to eating whatever they want.

While following the 16:8 method, you should also make sure that you drink plenty of water throughout the day, whether fasting or eating. This ensures that you don't become dehydrated and will also aid in digestion. Also, you should also exercise too!

Now, there are no rules to say that you must exercise while following an intermittent fasting routine, but it will help you lose weight faster, and it will help with your general health and wellbeing. Exercise is fantastic on so many levels, not least helping to build lean muscle, which also boosts your ability to burn fat as an energy source. Exercise is also known to help with mental health issues, such as anxiety and depression, as well as stress. We all live stressful lives, and a little exercise can sometimes be enough to reduce it extremely manageable levels. Aside from anything else, exercise can be a friendly and fun activity!

16/8 Method Step-by-Step

Now it's time to get into the real nitty-gritty of what this method entails.

We've mentioned that there are many different types of intermittent fasting, and some do ask you to fast for 24 hours a few times a week. The 16:8 method differs because there are no long and arduous fasts, you fast for 16 hours every day and normally eat for eight hours.

Now, 16 hours may sound like a lot, but you will be asleep for most of it.. We'll talk about how to follow the method in more detail, but a good example is someone who needs to eat breakfast versus someone who doesn't want to eat early in the mornings. We're all different, but most of us fall into one of these two categories. You might wake up starving and need breakfast otherwise, you can't focus, or you might wake up and simply need a coffee and feel a little sick if you eat straight away.

You can manage this two ways, just to give you an example of what the 16:8 method looks like.

If you need breakfast, you can eat it as soon as you wake up, kick-starting your eight-hour eating period. So if you wake up at 8:00 a.m., you have breakfast at 8:30 a.m., and that means you need to finish eating by 4:30 p.m. You might go to bed at 10:00 p.m., which means you're only consciously fasting 15.5 hours. As you can see, it's not as horrendous as it sounds, and you can drink water, non-calorie containing drinks, and unsweetened black tea or coffee during your fasting times too. I repeat again that it's actually highly recommended to drink plenty of water because dehydration is not something you want to play Russian roulette with.

The other scenario is that you are someone who don´t want to eat when they wake up. In this case, you can get up, get dressed, have a black, unsweetened coffee, and you can skip breakfast, starting your eating window at lunchtime. So, for instance, you would begin eating at 12:00 p.m. This means you can eat freely until

8:00 p.m. You would then perhaps sleep at 10:00 p.m., which means you're effectively not consciously fasting very much. This is why the 16:8 method is so popular and effective.

Of course, you need to be mindful of what you're eating during your eight-hour eating window. If you cram those eight hours full of chips and chocolate, then you're going to eat far more calories than you should in the full 24 hours of the day, and you'll probably gain weight rather than lose it! If, however, you're mindful of what you eat, not particularly being restrictive, but simply thinking more along the lines of health, you'll be full and satisfied by the end of your eating window and ready for your fast. This means you will lose weight quite easily and receive the overall benefits of intermittent fasting too.

What You Can Eat

Again, there are no rules on what you can eat and what you can't eat. It's a free choice when following the 16:8 diet. However, what you should be in mind is overall health and choices that are considered healthy, compared to unhealthy.

The idea is to create that calorie deficit during the full 24-hour span. You do this by ensuring that you fast and eat for the correct ratios of time: eight hours eating and 16 hours fasting, and that during your eating times, you stick to healthy options as much as possible.

If you want a few ideas on some of the healthiest foods you can incorporate into your day, check out the list below.

Eggs

Make sure you eat the yolk because this contains vitamins and protein.

Leafy Greens

We're talking about spinach, collards, kale, and Swiss chard, to name a few, and these are packed with fiber and are low in calories.

Oily and Fatty Fish, Such as Salmon

Salmon is a fish that will keep you feeling full, but it's also high in Omega-3 fatty acids, which are ideal for boosting brain health, reducing inflammation, and generally helping with weight loss too. If salmon isn't your bag, try mackerel, trout, herring, and sardines instead.

Cruciferous Vegetables

In this case, you need to look to Brussels sprouts, broccoli, cabbage, and cauliflower. Again, these types of vegetables contain a high fiber, which helps you feel fuller for longer, and have cancer-fighting attributes.

Lean Meats

Stick to beef and chicken for the best options, but make sure you go for the leanest cuts possible. You'll get a good protein boost here, but you can also make all manner of delicious dishes with both types of meat.

Boiled Potatoes

You might think that potatoes are bad for you, and in most cases, they are, especially if you fry them, but boiled potatoes are a good choice, particularly if you lack in potassium. They are also very filling.

Tuna

This is a different type of fish to the oily fish we mentioned earlier, and it's very low fat but high in protein. Go for tuna canned in water and not oil for the healthiest option. Pile it onto a jacket potato for a delicious and healthy meal.

Beans and Other Types of Legumes

These are the staple of any healthy diet and are super filling too. We're talking about kidney beans, lentils, and black beans here, and they're high in fiber and protein.

Cottage Cheese

If you're a cheese fan, there's no reason to deny yourself, but most cheeses are quite high in fat. In that case, why not opt for cottage cheese instead? This is high in protein and quite filling but low in calories.

Avocados

The fad food of the moment is very healthy and great for boosting your brainpower. Mash it up on some toast for a great breakfast packed with potassium and plenty of fiber.

Nuts

Instead of snacking on chocolate and chips, why not snack on nuts? You'll get great amounts of healthy fats, as well as fiber and protein, and they're filling too. But don't eat too many, as they can be high in calories if you overindulge.

Whole Grains

Everyone knows that whole grains are packed with fiber and therefore keep you fuller for longer, so this is the ideal choice for anyone who is trying intermittent fasting. Try quinoa, brown rice, and oats to get you started.

Fruits

Not all fruits are healthy, but they're certainly a better option than junk food. You'll also get a plethora of different vitamins and minerals, as well as a boost of antioxidants into your diet, ideal for your immune system.

Seeds

Again, just like nuts, seeds make a great snack, and they can be sprinkled on many foods, such as yogurt and porridge. Try chia seeds for a high fiber treat while being low calorie at the same time.

Coconut Oil

You will no doubt have heard of the wonders of coconut oil, and this is a very healthy oil to try cooking with. Coconut oil is made up medium-chain triglycerides, and while you might panic at the word triglycerides, these are the healthy kind.

Foods to Avoid

Fruit Juices

It is never advisable to have fruit juices. Fresh or packed, fruit juices are not good for your body. They raise your blood sugar levels instantly without adding fiber to your system. Drinking juice is like adding empty calories to your system.

Soda and Other Caloric Beverages

Like juices, they also add empty calories to your system. In addition, they are even worse for your body as they are prepared from refined sugar. You will start feeling cravings to have more soon after you have some.

Refined Flours

Refined flours and the products made from them are bad for your health. These flours do not have the original fiber content and are very easy to process. This means that after consuming refined flours, you will again start feeling hungry very soon. They are bad for your digestive system and raise your blood sugar levels very fast.

Sugar

Sugar in any form should be avoided. You must buy everything after checking the label. If it has sugar, maple syrup, fructose, or any other such thing at the top of the ingredient list, it must be avoided. Such things will make your fasting routine very difficult as you will have food cravings and frequent hunger pangs.

Processed Food

Processed food items are bad for your health. To increase the shelf life of processed food items, a lot of sugar is added to them. In place of healthy fats, trans fats and hydrogenated fats are used.

All these things are very bad for your health; hence, you must avoid them at all costs.

Trans Fats

Trans fats are bad, and although most processed food items don't have trans fat listed as an ingredient or its value is given as zero, it is not the whole truth. The best way is to avoid highly processed food items, especially the ones with a lot of added preservatives.

Managing the Macronutrients

There are 3 main components of any meal:

- Fat
- Protein
- Carbohydrate

You must consume all these macronutrients in a balanced manner. Having a nutrient-dense meal always helps curb hunger pangs for a long and suppresses the food cravings.

The ideal distribution of the macronutrients should be in the ratio given below:

Fat: 70-75%

Fat is dense, and the body takes a lot of time to process fats. This means that when you consume a fat-rich diet, it keeps you feeling full for longer and prevents hunger pangs. The body takes much longer in processing the fats, which also helps prevent the insulin spike in your body. You can easily get a lot of calories even by eating fat in small quantities. When you have to consume many calories in fewer meals, making fat the main component of your meal always helps.

However, you must ensure that you eat healthy fats. You can get healthy fats from animal meat, fish, nuts, seeds, and fruits. 1 gram of fat provides 9 calories. It is more than double the number of calories received from carbs of the same weight. This means you can get more calories by consuming fat in smaller quantities. You must include healthy fats in your diet to stay satiated.

Protein: 20-25%

Protein is essential for building muscles. When your body is running on a low-carb diet, and you are doing a lot of exercises, there is a loss of muscle mass. The muscles are constantly breaking, and new ones are building. To help this process, you will need to consume a lot of protein. Therefore, protein should form the second biggest part of your meals. However, you should never consume protein in excess as that would again get broken as glucose.

You can get protein from lean meats, fish, nuts, dairy, egg white, and legumes.

Carbohydrate: 5-10%

Carbohydrates should constitute the smallest part of your meal. You must not consume refined carbs as they get processed very quickly and increase blood sugar levels. However, once the body processes the refined carbs, you would start feeling hungry again. Consumption of refined carbs would lead to food cravings and hunger pangs.

Typical Schedule for the 16/8 Method

Early Eating Schedule

This schedule is a great option because it takes advantage of your circadian rhythm. It's also the ideal time to eat because it avoids binging at night. However, it means that you're going to eat an early dinner, which might not work for everyone. With this schedule, you'll start eating at 7:00 a.m. and end at 3:00 p.m.

Here is how to ease into your fast:

Time	Days 1–3	Days 4–6	Days 7–9	Days 10–12
7:00 a.m.	Wake up Eat	Wake up Eat	Wake up Eat	Wake up Eat
9:00 a.m.				
11:00 a.m.	Eat	Eat	Eat	Eat
1:00 p.m.				
3:00 p.m.	Snack		Eat	Eat before 3:00
5:00 p.m.		Eat	Fast	Fast
7:00 p.m.	Eat	Fast	Fast	Fast
9:00 p.m.	Fast	Fast	Fast	Fast
10:00 p.m.	Sleep/fast	Sleep/fast	Sleep/fast	Sleep/fast

Here is your weeklong schedule once you've eased into the fast:

Time	12:00 a.m.– 7:00 a.m.	7:00 a.m.	11:00 a.m.	2:00 p.m.	3:00 p.m.– 2:00 a.m.
Monday to Sunday	Fast/sleep	Breakfast (either light or the largest meal of the day)	Large meal	Last meal, finished by 3:00 p.m.	Fast/sleep

Midday Eating Schedule

Some people have difficulty with eating first thing in the morning. In this case, you can start your fast later in the day. This fast is ideal for people who want to eat right in the middle of the day

Here is how to ease into your fast:

Time	Days 1–3	Days 4–6	Days 7–9	Days 10–12
6:00 a.m.	Sleep/eat	Sleep/east	Sleep/fast	Sleep/fast
8:00 a.m.	Eat	Eat	Eat	Fast
10:00 a.m.				Eat
12:00 p.m.	Eat	Eat	Eat	
2:00 p.m.	Snack	Snack		Eat
4:00 p.m.				
6:00 p.m.	Eat	Eat	Eat	Eat before 6:00 p.m.
8:00 p.m.			Fast	Fast
10:00 p.m.	Sleep/fast	Sleep/fast	Sleep/fast	Sleep/fast

Here is your weeklong schedule once you've eased into the fast:

Time	12:00 a.m.– 7:00 a.m.	10:00 a.m.	2:00 p.m.	5:00 p.m.	6:00 p.m.– 12:00 a.m.
Monday to Sunday	Fast/sleep	Breakfast (either light or the largest meal of the day)	Large meal	Last meal, finished by 6:00 p.m.	Fast/sleep

Evening Eating Schedule

This schedule doesn't take advantage of your circadian rhythm, and it might not give you the most benefits in changing glucose and cortisol levels. However, this schedule can work for people who appreciate social eating or work at unconventional hours. You can always eat a bit earlier to change this schedule.

Here is how to ease into your fast:

Time	Days 1–3	Days 4–6	Days 7–9	Days 10–12
12:00 a.m.– 6:00 a.m.	Sleep/fast	Sleep/fast	Sleep/fast	Sleep/fast
8:00 a.m.	Fast	Fast	Fast	Fast
10:00 a.m.	Eat	Fast	Fast	Fast
12:00 p.m.		Eat	Fast	Fast
2:00 p.m.	Eat		Eat	Fast
4:00 p.m.	Snack	Eat	Snack	Eat
6:00 p.m.		Snack		
8:00 p.m.	Eat		Eat	Eat
10:00 p.m.		Eat		
12:00 a.m.			Eat	Eat before midnight

Here is your weeklong schedule once you've eased into the fast:

Time	12:00 a.m.– 8:00 a.m.	8:00 a.m.– 4:00 p.m.	4:00 p.m.	8:00 p.m.	11:00 p.m.– 12:00 a.m.
Monday to Sunday	Fast/sleep	Fast	Breakfast (either light or the largest meal of the day)	Large meal	Last meal, finished by midnight

These three different schedules give you some options for following your 16/8 fasting schedule. As mentioned before, adapt the schedules to fit your own daily rhythm and lifestyle better. It's ideal if your schedule is consistent, but it doesn't have to be set in stone. If you know you want to celebrate your best friend's promotion at the end of the week, then shift your fasting schedule to accommodate eating with your friends. Remember, fasting isn't a diet; it's just an eating schedule. It doesn't need to be permanent, and there shouldn't be any guilt about shifting your schedule. Since we've now discussed several schedule possibilities and how to ease into them, we'll spend the next couple of chapters looking at food choices and some meal plans.

Does IF Have Different Effects on Men and Women?

No one is stating ladies are more sensitive than men. In any case, it's conceivable that irregular fasting unexpectedly influences people. We could do with much more research right now no methods is this a sweeping speculation; many men despise fasting, and a lot of ladies blossom with it. There is proof to recommend that ladies may be increasingly vulnerable to negative impacts.

The procedure is profoundly directed in ladies as it's engaged with ovulation, dependent on cycles and calendars. It's conceivable that among ladies, gonadotropin discharging hormone is all the more effortlessly upset by changes to one's propensities and routines, so skirting one's typical supper can some of the time cause more uneasiness among ladies than men. Ladies have been appeared to have a more significant level of a protein called kisspeptin, which makes it more noteworthy to fasting. While more research is should have been done on this, it bodes well to coherently reason that the hormonal move (from fasting) can influence digestion.

Chapter 4: Scientific Facts About Intermittent Fasting

Intermittent fasting has been found to help people lose weight and also promote their health. However, conventional calorie restrictions diets are superior to IF. This is according to a study called **HELENA**- intermittent fasting's largest research in history. It was done by scientists from Heidelberg University Hospital and the German Cancer Research Center (DKFZ). They found out that there are different routes to achieve a healthier weight. You have to get a diet plan that suits you best.

Increased Brain Cell Production

This is one of the most surprising yet amazing benefits of intermittent fasting. Fasting has been shown to enhance neurogenesis, which develops new brain cells and nerves. Optimizing the brain's neurogenesis can help to improve your mood, focus, memory, and other cognitive functions.

One study published in the Journal of Cerebral Blood Flood and Metabolism shows that mice that fasted produced more brain cells than mice on a regular diet. The researchers measured cell production, cell death, and neurogenesis. Following 3 months of intermittent fasting, the mice that fasted showed increased brain cells and had less brain cell damage from a stroke.

Research shows that fasting may positively affect your brain as exercise has on your body. These activities place stress on the brain, making it stronger and more resistant to stressful stimuli. The brain reacts to stressful stimuli by building up new neurons and connections.

Both exercise and fasting seem to boost ketones and mitochondria production within the brain. Also, new neural connections and synapses are created and strengthened. This leads to better memory and learning.

Increased BDNF Production

Besides promoting neurogenesis, fasting increases brain-derived neurotrophic factor (BDNF). BDNF is a growth factor and is critical for cognitive function. BDNF produces new brain cells and nerves and creates connections between them. It also helps with learning and memory and is a natural antidepressant. Higher levels of BDNF keep neurons healthy and ensures the neurons communicate effectively with one another. In contrast, lower levels of BDNF can increase the risks of memory loss, dementia, and other cognitive problems.

According to a study by Bronwen Martin, Mark P. Mattson, and Stuart Maudsley (2006), fasting for 16 to 18 hours can increase BDNF production by 100 %, and fasting for 36 hours can increase BDNF production by as much 400 %.

Other research by the National Institute on Aging in the U.S. has shown that mice who fasted every other day showed improvements in their cognitive functioning. The researchers team put 40 mice on an alternate day fasting schedule (one day on, one day off) and noted that the parts of their brain responsible for memory were more active.

Besides, the brain protein, brain-derived neurotrophic factor (BDNF), increased by up to 50 percent in the mice that fasted.

May Protect Against Alzheimer's

Alzheimer's is a dementia type that slowly destroys memory and mental functions over time. Currently, there isn't a cure for Alzheimer's. One study looked at whether intermittent fasting improved the cognitive function of people with Alzheimer's. Researchers looked at ten people with early signs of Alzheimer's. Each person was asked to make some lifestyle modifications, including fasting for 12 hours each night. 6 months later, 9 out of the 10 subjects showed improvements in their cognitive abilities.

How Intermittent Fasting Impacts Human Growth Hormone (HGH))

When you fast, your HGH levels go up. This helps to preserve lean muscle and breaks down fat. When free fatty acids are released and converted into energy, this process is known as lipolysis.

Obese individuals generally have inefficient lipolysis processes. Lower HGH levels may be one possible cause of this.

Besides fasting, HGH levels can also be increased by exercise. These levels can fluctuate throughout the day since the pituitary gland releases the HGH hormone in spurts. Our HGH levels are generally higher when we wake up. We produce growth hormone during sleep, which increases our blood glucose that can be used as fuel for the day. Thus, this idea that you have to eat breakfast to get energy is false. Your body is already primed and ready to function in the morning without having to load up on food.

In addition, many popular breakfast choices, such as cereals and toasts, are high in sugar and carbs. This can make you feel tired and lethargic.

HGH is a natural testosterone booster and has been shown to increase muscle strength and improve exercise performance. Many bodybuilders and athletes may inject additional HGH to improve their performance. A study by the International Journal of Endocrinology looked at the effects of HGH on muscle strength in men over 50 years old. 14 healthy male subjects were divided into two groups: seven subjects were placed in the HGH therapy group, while the remaining seven were placed in the placebo group. 6 months later, all the participants were tested for their body composition and muscle strength, including some exercises, such as the leg press and bench press exercises. The HGH group showed a significant increase in muscle strength in the lower body than the placebo group.

One study by the Journal of Clinical Investigation showed that intermittent fasting dramatically increased men's growth hormone production.

Another research from the Journal of Clinical Endocrinology and Metabolism showed intermittent fasting reduced leptin levels in obese adults. This led to instantaneous increases in testosterone levels.

A fascinating study by the European Journal of Endocrinology showed that fasting dramatically increased the Gonadotropin-Releasing Hormone (GnRH), a testosterone precursor, in both obese and non-obese men. The researchers looked at 17 men divided into two groups (9 men in the obese group and 8 men in the non-obese group). GnRH levels in the obese men rose by 26% while the GnRH levels in non-obese men rose by 67%. In addition, serum testosterone levels shot up by 180% in those in the non-obese group.

Fasting and Leptin

Fasting is one way to increase leptin and glucose sensitivity. Leptin levels have been shown to fall after a short-term fast and return to normal after eating. Any form of fasting should work since it forces the body to burn through excess glucose stores.

A study published in the Journal of Clinical Endocrinology & Metabolism looked at how fasting affected nine obese men's leptin levels. After three days of fasting, the researchers noted that the subjects had reductions in total body mass (21.4 ± 3.7%) and leptin (76.3 ± 8.1%). Leptin levels returned to baseline levels within 12 hours of eating.

Another study published in Metabolism looked at the changes in serum leptin and endocrine in both men and women after 7 days of fasting. The subjects were made up of 11 men and 13 women. After 7 days of fasting, the researchers noted that both men and women lost an average of 4 percent in body weight. Leptin decreased in both men (from 3.7 ± 0.5 to 2.1 ± 0.4 ng/mL) and women (16.2 ± 1.9 ng/mL to 6.0 ± 0.8 ng/mL) following fasting. Compared to men, women had higher levels of leptin before and after calorie restriction. However, women showed a bigger decrease in leptin levels overall.

As these studies show, fasting seems to effectively reduce leptin levels and body mass in both men and women.

Fasting and Inflammation?

There is proof that intermittent fasting may be an effective way to reduce inflammation. Research shows that intermittent fasting may have a protective effect against high blood pressure, high insulin, and inflammation. Evidence shows that fasting may help with type 2 diabetes and autoimmune conditions like MS and rheumatoid arthritis.

In a study published by the National Center for Biotechnology Information, researchers fed mice either a low-fat or high-fat diet for 10-12 weeks. After fasting, the mice fed a low-fat diet lost more body weight (18% compared to 5%), performed better on memory and learning tasks, and showed better locomotor activity than the mice on a high-fat diet. Low-fat mice also had an improved nervous system and immune function. The researchers concluded that fasting has an anti-inflammatory effect on the neuroimmune system, which a high-fat diet prevents.

Ramadan fasting has been shown to to affect reducing inflammation and may even help treat fatty liver. One study published in the US National Library of Medicine in 2017 compared 83 people with Nonalcoholic fatty liver disease (NAFLD), 42 who fasted, and 41 controls who didn't fast for Ramadan. Those who fasted showed significant reductions in glucose, plasma insulin, insulin resistance, and inflammation compared to the non-fasting group.

Chapter 5: Exercise and Fasting

Exercising is important as it helps in burning fat faster. It is also essential for building healthier muscles. All those who have been objecting exercise in a fasted state only explain one side of the story.

There are a few things on which everyone agrees:

- Exercises help in burning fat

- They help in keeping the body fit

- They also help in uplifting your mood and bringing positivity

Some experts believe that when you exercise in the fasted state, your body feels the energy crunch and tries to break muscles as calories. This will happen because, after carbs end, the muscles are the easiest form of energy. The muscles are made of protein, and protein can also be broken down easily. However, it isn't that simple.

Although it is correct that some muscle loss takes place while you are doing exercise, it is wrong to assume that it happens because your body is trying to produce energy from them. Some loss of muscle mass would occur even after you have had a high dose of glucose drink. This happens because the muscles are continuously getting damaged during exercise, and they break apart to give way to stronger ones.

Once your body has exhausted the glucose and glycogen reserves, it starts burning the fat reserves for energy. The fat is a more reliable and long-lasting energy source, and it can fulfill all the body's energy needs without causing any harm. To think that the body would think or behave otherwise is irrational.

Exercising is the key to living healthy, and if you're choosing to fast for the same reason, it makes sense that you'll want to add exercise to your fasting schedule. This isn't a requirement for having a successful fast, but many people already exercise before fasting and want to continue it. Whether you're just starting with exercise or you want to continue your normal workout routine.

When to Exercise

Fasting is all about when to eat, even more so than what to eat. The importance of timing is what helps you become the healthiest. So, on that health journey, the timing of exercise should be taken into consideration. This is a question that many people have when first doing intermittent fasting. Most of us believe that if we don't have food, then we'll end up shaky and weak while we exercise. Some people may indeed feel like this, but some people are completely fine with exercising without eating first. Let's investigate the different options for when to exercise.

Exercising Before You Eat

There are many people who choose to exercise early in the morning before they head to work. Many of them exercise during a fasted state, where they haven't eaten after they woke up. To them, they may feel that they perform better without food in their stomach. But what about if you're fasting for 16 hours before you exercise? Is this a healthy way to exercise? Well, yes and no.

There is a lot of conflicting research and information about whether someone should exercise in a fasted state. In some studies, there were results where people burned more stores of fat. This was more than if they had eaten before fasting. You may burn more fat because there isn't any intake to fuel your workout. So, while your body might normally have recently ingested carbs to burn, the body can only use its stores of fat when exercising in a fasted state. While this sounds really promising, it doesn't add anything to your exercise. You're not going to lose more weight or more fat; it's just that your body is using its stores quicker. The benefit that you will receive is better blood sugar levels since you won't have anything ingested to mess with them.

There are some downsides to fasting and exercising without eating. These are not always supported in research, but there is a chance that your body will burn through your muscle protein instead of your fat stores to provide fuel. This means that you'll lose muscle mass as your body uses it to get through the workout.

This is negative because it does the exact opposite of what a workout is supposed to do. There's also another negative aspect, which is that exercising on a fast may slow down your metabolism. So, when choosing your exercise time, take into consideration some of these possible drawbacks.

Exercising After You Eat

The other option is to exercise after you eat. Many people like to do this because they may feel dizzy or weak if they exercise on an empty stomach. Eating before you exercise has long been proven to be beneficial, especially for athletes who need the energy to keep exercising for hours. Eating a carb-heavy meal before you do a long-duration exercise can provide your body with the needed energy and glucose to power your workout without you feeling weak. They'll help strengthen you. However, most of us aren't athletes. So, do we need to eat before we exercise? It just depends on you.

Go with What Makes You Comfortable

The best choice for figuring out your workout times while fasting is to go with whatever makes you feel the most comfortable. As mentioned earlier, some people feel weak if they don't eat before they work out. Some people feel nauseous if they exercise after eating, even after several hours of eating. So, choose the time that works best for you.

The reason why you can choose your own timing because, through all the research studies on exercising in a fasted or non-fasted state, researchers couldn't find consistent results that showed one was better than the other. The research isn't consistent, and most of them demonstrate no difference between whether you eat before or after you exercise.

If you're still not sure which way to go, then break it down like this:

• If you're going to do short-duration training or a low-impact exercise, then you don't have to eat before you exercise.

• If you're going to do a high-duration exercise or a high-impact exercise, then eat three to four hours before you plan on exercising.

Either way, once you are finished exercising, you should eat something. It doesn't have to be immediately, but it should be as soon as you can. Eating after exercising helps your body recover by giving it the necessary protein and carbs to build up its stores again. If you're exercising right before your eating window, then have a good meal once you are finished. At that point, you would have been without food for 16 hours and would have just used up the last of your stores of energy. So, eat a good meal to help you recover faster.

Exercising on Different Fasting Schedules

Based on which fasting schedule you choose to follow, there are several different options of when to exercise. It's best not to exercise after your last meal in the evening unless you couldn't get it in earlier. While you are transitioning into your fasting schedule, ease up on your normal workout routine. Your body is already going through a change, and keeping your same workout (or starting a new one while also starting your fast) may cause you some discomfort. Once you've settled into your fasting schedule, you can start exercising again at your regular level or start a new exercise routine.

For the early eating schedule and assuming you wake up at 6:00 a.m., you could exercise between 6:00 a.m. and 7:00 a.m. Since you'll be exercising in a fast state, work with some exercises that are low-impact and in short duration. Consider something like yoga, biking, or walking for less than an hour. You could even do some light weightlifting. After exercising, eat your first meal of the day at 7:00 a.m. Make sure that your first meal is substantial and has a good mix of protein and fiber.

For the other fasting schedules, you can follow the same information. So, for the midday eating schedule, you could start exercising at 9:00 a.m. and break your fast at 10:00 a.m. For the evening eating schedule, exercise between 3:00 p.m. and 4:00

p.m. Break your fast at 4:00 p.m. with a meal that is high in protein and fiber.

Here's one final note about exercising in a fasted state: If you're used to exercising in a fasted state, then make sure you take some time to adjust to your new fasting time. It's important to recognize that you've just spent 16 hours fasting, which is significantly different from exercising after eight hours of sleep.

If you want to exercise after eating, you would exercise three hours after your morning meal or three hours after your midday meal then during the early eating schedule. You'll follow the same pattern for the other eating schedules. Whichever you choose, make sure that you can eat after you exercise. Don't exercise at the end of your eating window when you can't eat. Since you'll have a meal before you exercise at this time, you can do high-intensity exercise or endurance exercise. This includes things like playing a game of basketball, long-distance running, or HIIT workouts.

Chapter 6: Different Methods of IF

Lean-Gains Method

This intermittent fasting method focuses on a healthy diet, fasting, and rigorous exercises. It is popular because of its ability to convert fats straight to muscle. The main objective of this method is to fast 14-16 hours every day from when you wake up.

Waking up and fasting up to 1 pm and doing a warmup and stretches just before midday is a perfect approach to this method. From midday, do any exercise of choice for up to one hour and break your fast at 1 pm.

From there, go about your day's activities normally, and when it is around 4pm, eat again. Eat again at around 9 pm. This will give you about 15hours of fast until 1 pm on the following day. If it is challenging at the beginning, you can start fasting for 13 hours for several days and then increasing to 15 hours.

14:10 Method

In this method, you fast for 14 hours and eat during the other 100 hours. It works similarly way as the 16:8. The difference is that the eating period in this method is 10 hours, instead of 8 hours in 14:8.

20:4 Method

Whereas 14:10 method was an easier step down from 16:8 method, 20:4 method is absolutely an increase in terms of difficulty. It's a more intense method certainly, for it requires 20 hours of fasting within each day with only a 4-hour eating window for the individual to gain all their nutrients and energy.

The majority of the people who opt to use this method end up having either one large meal with several snacks or two smaller meals with fewer snacks. 20:4 is flexible in that sense—the sense whereby the individual chooses how the eating window is divided amongst meals and snacks.

20:4 method is tricky, for many people instinctually overeat during the eating window, but that's neither necessary nor is it healthy. People who choose 20:4 method should try to keep meal portions around the same size that they normally have been without fasting. Experimenting on how many snacks are needed will be helpful as well with this method.

Many people end up working up to 20:4 from other methods, based on what their bodies can handle and what they're ready to attempt. Few start with 20:4, so if it's not working for you right away, please don't be too hard on yourself! Step it back to 16:8, and then see how soon you can get back to where you'd like to be.

The Warrior Method

The warrior method is quite similar to the 20:4 method in that the individual fasts for 20 hours within each day and breaks fast for a 4-hour eating window. The difference is in the outlook and mindset of the practitioner, however. Essentially, the thought process behind the warrior method is that, in ancient times, the hunter coming home from stalking prey or the warrior coming home from battle would really only get one meal each day. One meal would have to provide sustenance for the rest of the day, recuperative energy from the ordeal, and sustainable energy for the future.

Therefore, practitioners of the warrior method are encouraged to have one large meal when they breakfast, and that meal should be jam-packed with fats, proteins, and carbs for the rest of the day (and for the days ahead). Just like with the 20:4 method, however, it can sometimes be too intense for practitioners, and it's very easy to scale this one back in forcefulness by making up a method like 18:6 or 17:7. If it's not working, don't force it to work past two weeks, but do try to make it through a week to see if it's your stubbornness or if it's just a mismatch with the method.

12:12 Method

12:12 method is a little easier, along with the lines of 14:10, rather than 16:8 or 20:4. Beginners to Intermittent Fasting would do well to try this one right off the bat. Some people get 12 hours of sleep each night and can easily wake up from the fasting period, ready to engage with the eating window. Many people use this method in their lives without even knowing it.

To go about 12:12 method in your life, however, you'll want to be as purposeful about it as you can be. Make sure to be strict about your 12-hour cut-offs. Make sure it's working and feeling good in your body, and then you're invited to take things up a notch and try, say, 14:10 or maybe your invention, like 15:11. Always, start with what works and then move up (or down) to what feels right (and even possibly better).

5:2 Method

5:2 method is popular among those who want to take things up a notch generally. Instead of fasting and eating within each day, these individuals practice fasting two whole days out of the week. The other 5 days are free to eat, exercise, or diet as desired, but those other two days (which can be consecutive or scattered throughout the week) must be strictly fasting days.

For those fasting days, it's not as if the individual can't eat anything altogether, however. In actuality, one can consume no more than 500 calories each day for this Intermittent Fasting method. I suppose these fasting days would be better referred to as "restricted-intake" days, for that is a more accurate description.

5:2 method is advantageous, but it is also one of the more difficult ones to attempt. If that works better for you, don't be ashamed to embrace it! However, if you're dedicated to having days "on" and days "off" with fasting and eating, there are other alternatives, too.

Eat-Stop-Eat (24-Hour) Method

The eat-stop-eat or 24-hour method is another option for people who want to have days "on" and "off" between fasting and eating. It's a little less intense than the 5:2 method, and it's much more flexible for the person, depending on what he or she needs. For instance, if you need a literal 24-hour fast each week and that's it, you can do that. Meanwhile, if you want a more flexible 5:2 method-type thing to happen, you can work with what you want and create a method surrounding those desires and goals.

The most successful approaches to the eat-stop-eat method have involved more strict dieting (or at the very least, cautious and healthy eating) during the 5 or 6 days when the individual engages in the week's free-eating window. For the individual to truly see success with weight loss, there will have to be some caloric restriction (or high nutrition focus) those 5 or 6 days, too, so that the body will have a version of consistency in health and nutrition content.

On the one or two days each week the individual decides to fast, there can still be highly-restricted caloric intake. As with the 5:2

method, he or she can consume no more than 500 calories worth of food and drink during these fasting days so that the body can maintain energy flow and more.

If the individual engages in exercise, those workout days should absolutely be reserved for the 5 or 6 free-eating days. The same goes for the 5:2 method. Try not to exercise (at least not excessively) on those days that are chosen for fasting. Your body will not appreciate the added stress when you're taking in so few calories. As always, you can choose to move up from eat-stop-eat to another method if this works easily and you're interested in something more. Furthermore, you can start with a strict 24-hour method and then move up to a more flexible eat-stop-eat approach! Do what feels right, and never be afraid to troubleshoot one method for the sake of choosing another.

Alternate-Day Method

The alternate-day method is similar to the eat-stop-eat and 5:2 methods because it focuses on individual days "on" and "off" for fasting and eating. The difference for this method, in particular, is that it ends up being at least 2 days a week fasting, and sometimes, it can be as many as 4.

Some people follow very strict approaches to the alternate-day method and literally fast every other day, only consuming 500 calories or less on those days designated for fasting. On the other hand, some people are much more flexible, and they tend to go for two days eating, one day fasting, two days eating, one day fasting, _etc._ The alternate-day method is even more flexible than eat-stop-eat in that sense, for it allows the individual to choose how he or she alternates between eating and fasting, based on what works for the body and mind the best.

This more intense fasting style works particularly well for people who are working on equally intense fitness regimens, surprisingly. People who are eating more calories a day than 2000 (which is true for many bodybuilders and fitness buffs) will have more to gain from the alternate-day method, for you only have to cut back your eating on fasting days to about 25% of your standard caloric intake. Therefore, those fasting days can still provide solid nutritional support for fitness experts while helping them sculpt their bodies and maintain a new level of health.

Spontaneous Skipping Method

Alternate-day method and eat-stop-eat method are certainly flexible in their approaches to when the individual fasts and when he or she eats. However, none of those mentioned above plans are quite as flexible as the spontaneous skipping method. The spontaneous skipping method only requires that the individual skip meals within each day, whenever desired (and when it's sensed that the body can handle it).

Many people with more sensitive digestive systems or who practice more intense fitness regimens will start their experiences with IF through the spontaneous skipping method before moving on to something more intensive. People who have very haphazard daily schedules or people around food a lot but forget to eat will benefit from this method, for it works well with chaotic schedules and unplanned energies.

Despite that chaotic and unorganized potential, the spontaneous skipping method can also be more structured and organized, depending on what you make of it! For instance, someone desiring more structure can choose which meal each day they'd like to skip. Let's say he chooses to skip breakfast each day. Then, his spontaneous skipping method will be structured around making sure to skip breakfast (a.k.a.—not to eat until at least 12 pm) daily. Whatever you need to do to make this method work, try it! This method is made for experimentation and adventurousness.

Crescendo Method

The method is very well-suited for female practitioners (since their anatomies can be so detrimental to high-intensity fasts). This approach is essentially made for internal awareness, gentle introductions, and gradual additions, depending on what works and what doesn't. It's a very active, trial-and-error type of method.

The individual starts by only fasting 2 or 3 days a week through crescendo method, and on those fast days, it wouldn't be a very intense fast at all. It wouldn't even be so strict that the individual would have to consume no more than 500 calories, like with 5:2, eat-stop-eat, and others. Instead, these "fasting" days would be trial periods for methods like 12:12, 14:10, 16:8, or 20:4. The remaining 4 or 5 days out of the week would be open eating-window periods, but again, the practitioner is encouraged to maintain a healthy diet throughout the week.

The crescendo method works extremely well for female practitioners because it enables them to see how methods like 14:10 or 12:12 will affect their bodies without tying them to the method hook, line, and sinker. It allows them to see what each method does to their hormone levels, menstruation tendencies, and mood swings. Therefore, the crescendo method encourages these people to be more in touch with their bodies before moving too quickly into something that could do serious anatomical and hormonal damage.

Crescendo method will work extremely well for overweight or diabetic practitioners, too, for it will allow them to have these same "trial period" moments with all the methods before choosing what feels and works best, based on each situation.

Chapter 7: Tips and Tricks for Staying Healthy

Find a fasting buddy

It is easier to keep going when you know there is someone else fasting with you. It can be your husband, best friend, or family member. Sit down with them and walk them through the basics of the intermittent fasting technique you have chosen. Use each other as support on those days when one of you doesn't feel like fasting or exercising. It will be more fun when you have someone with who you can plan meals, shop for food, and learn.

Set Achievable Goals

It is best to start with short-term goals that you know you can achieve. Once you attain that goal, reward yourself, but don't do it with junk food. This will help boost your momentum and motivation.

Keep a Progress Journal

This is a great way to look at the positive changes you have experienced ever since you started your fast. Get a diary and start writing how you feel and all the progress you are making. It is essential to take time to look at how your body and life is transforming. Look at how your clothes fit, the energy you now have to play with your kids, and the way your sleep has improved. Track your positive progress and whip out that journal whenever you feel yourself losing motivation.

Don't Beat Yourself Up

Yes, there are days when you will fail and succumb to temptation. Things will get rough, and you will grab a cookie and start munching away. Be compassionate with yourself. Don't start talking negatively about yourself just because you didn't do things right.

Pray and Meditate

When you start to feel discouraged, take some time to feed and strengthen your soul and spirit. Pray, read scriptures, and meditate. This will help you love yourself despite the challenges you face in life.

Focus on the Good

I'm betting that you've found yourself with more energy throughout the first few weeks, especially following the feeding phase, had heightened alertness, euphoria, and even creativity. That felt great, didn't it? You've likely also had more time on your hands recently, particularly so if you are skipping a meal that you usually would spend a bit of time preparing.

Go Slow

These changes take a while, and they do not happen overnight. If you want to lose weight and make sure that it stays at bay, you'll need to slowly lose weight. You can starve yourself and shed a few pounds, but it will not do you any good. The more gradual and steadier your weight loss, the easier it is to maintain. Intermittent fasting is a great dieting option, and it is sustainable. Make sure you go slowly. There is no hurry, and you don't need to jump right in.

Be Your Coach

You are the best person to motivate yourself. You can program your mind to think precisely what you want it to think. You need to drive yourself by positively reinforcing your efforts and reminding yourself of your motivational reasons. Each day, you can program your mind and body to become an incredible fat-burning machine. When you use these self-motivational methods, your brain will believe everything you tell yourself.

Be Willing to Forgive Yourself

Don't forget, Intermittent Fasting is not a walk in the park. You may realize it's not as easy as people make it out to be. Perhaps you choose to attend a birthday party, and in the process, you ate delicious food instead of sticking to your fasting schedule. That's fine. Just remember, do not beat yourself up about it because this is normal, and you're only human. Instead of punishing yourself, realize the mistake, and immediately get back on track and move forward.

Setbacks Are Common

Temptation can strike, and there will be times when you might give in to your lures. After all, you are only human. It is okay to face a setback, but don't think of it as a failure. The attitude with which you deal with a delay can set the course for the rest of your diet.

Be Patient

One of the significant obstacles to a diet is the weight loss plateau. You might eat right and exercise correctly, but the numbers on the scales don't seem to change. The scale appears to be stuck for some reason. Well, this is known as the weight-loss plateau, and it is something that every dieter faces. Merely turn around and congratulate yourself on your success so far. It is a part of the process of weight loss.

Reward Yourself

Dieting does take some effort, and it might not seem fun at times. So, don't forget to treat yourself when you achieve a goal. A goal could be big or small. When you reach your goal, you should treat yourself. The reward doesn't have to be an extravagant one. Perhaps you can buy yourself a bottle of nail polish that you wanted! The rewards you set for yourself should never be food-related. Don't reward yourself with a pint of ice cream for losing 5 pounds in ten days. It doesn't make any sense and renders the diet redundant. When you celebrate your success, it will make you feel better about yourself and your food. It will also provide you with the necessary motivation to keep going even when you want to give up.

Incorporating Food Planning

Once you've got the basics down, planning your meals will help keep you on track and discourage you from looking for unhealthy food in periods of hunger. Research shows that people who plan their meals experience greater progress in their health and nutrition objectives and also save time and money in the end. As you get into the rhythm of intermittent fasting and your new way of life, you will make adjustments to your diet and your schedule.

Set Your Goals

Before you decide to start a diet, it is time to analyze why you want to start a diet. What are the reasons why you wish to diet? What are your goals? You might want to lose weight, improve your fitness levels, or even lead a healthier life. Reasons tend to vary from one individual to another. If you don't set any goals for yourself, you will quickly lose motivation after a couple of weeks of dieting. However, while setting goals. There are a couple of simple things you must keep in mind. Ensure that the goals you set are specific, measurable, attainable, relevant, and time-bound. Even if one of these ingredients is missing, then the chances of attaining such a goal will reduce.

Meal Plan

To ensure that you stick to the diet, you will need a meal plan. The good news is you don't have to create a meal plan for yourself. There is a detailed meal plan in this book. You can use it to get started with your new diet. Ensure that you include plenty of variety whenever you plan, the meals out for a week. If the food you eat starts getting repetitive, you will quickly lose interest to stick to your diet. Also, when you have a meal plan in place, it becomes easier to shop for groceries. If you know that you have a healthy meal waiting for you at home, the temptation of eating out will also reduce.

Make Calories Count

A common reason why a lot of people lose interest in dieting is because of hunger pangs. Ensure that you make every calorie count. Don't binge on unhealthy foods and instead, opt for nutrient-dense options. When your tummy is full, the urge to snack on junk food will reduce. If your daily calorie intake is 1800 calories, then ensure that you manage to eat at least two well-balanced, hearty meals. You can undoubtedly blow this calorie count by binging on a pint of ice cream, but it will do you no good.

Grocery Shopping

It is time to clean your pantry! Raid your kitchen and discard any unhealthy foods you find. Get rid of all cookies, cakes, chocolates, sodas, and other foods you must not eat while on the keto diet. Out of sight and out of mind is the best policy when it comes to dieting. If temptations surround you, the urge to give in will increase. Instead, stock up your pantry will keto-friendly ingredients. Once you have all the ingredients you need, it becomes easier to cook as well. Always prepare a grocery list before you go shopping and stick to this list.

Visualization

Whenever you are running low on motivation, remind yourself of the reasons why you started dieting. Think about the goals you want to attain. Start visualizing your goals. Think about how wonderful and happy you will feel when you attain your goals. While doing this, also think about how disappointed you would be if you didn't attain those same goals. While visualizing your goals, try to make the visualization as detailed as you possibly can. If you want, you can create a visualization board for yourself. Take a sheet of paper, note your goal on it, and place it somewhere visible. Glance at it daily. It will act as a subconscious reminder for your mind. Fill this board up with positive affirmations, quotes, or even images that motivate you to stick to the diet.

Start Gradually

When embarking on a new lifestyle or grappling with intermittent fasting, the food advice is to do it gradually. Everybody needs time to adapt and transition itself without haste. For instance, if you are fasting through the normal dinner time until six in the morning, make sure you see yourself through without any food around, even the ensuing day, even stretching up to lunchtime.

Physical Activity

Like meal planning, measuring foods, reading food labels, and portion control, exercise is NOT required, but beneficial to your overall results while doing intermittent fasting. The American Heart Association recommends some form of physical activity for at least 30 minutes daily.

Create a workout schedule. Make a leg day, an arms day, cardio day, total body weight day, and more. A schedule starts to make you more consistent and accountable. On days when you feel unmotivated to do one, you have the other. If you are already exercising, intermittent fasting can only improve your results. The combination of intermittent fasting and exercise maximizes weight loss and weight maintenance.

Mindset

The biggest barrier, if any, will be your mindset. The barrier will be the already set attitudes and assumptions you have in your head, specifically related to the relationship you have with food and eating food. Think mind over matter, and you matter the most to yourself, so take better care of yourself. To sustain following an intermittent lifestyle, you will need to erase or ignore all prior assumptions or attitudes related to diets/lifestyle changes, losing weight, current food habits, current eating schedules, changes in general, and more. Once started, try to make optimal choices for yourself and be disciplined in carrying out your plans. To be successful, you will need to think and act differently for optimal results.

Take Photos and Measurements

If weight reduction is one of your objectives, don't depend entirely on the scale. Your real weight can vary fundamentally from every day, and you probably won't see enormous changes in the numbers in any event, when your body is experiencing a massive change. You can utilize the scale as an instrument, yet take these everyday numbers while considering others factors. Rather, take "before" and "after" (or "progress") pictures. Pictures can be truly motivating tools. When you see yourself consistently, you may not see the little changes happening, however, when you analyze pictures taken a month, the progressions might be fundamentally increasingly obvious. Try not to let any present disappointment with your body prevent you from taking before pictures. You'll be glad you have them not far off. Notwithstanding pictures, it's useful to take body measurement.

Chapter 8: Recipes

Breakfast

#1 Onion Tofu

Preparation Time: 8 min - **Cooking Time**: 5 min - **Servings**: 3

Ingredients:

- 2 blocks tofu, pressed and cubed into 1-inch pieces

- 2 medium onions, sliced

- 2 tbsp. butter

- 1 cup cheddar cheese, grated

- salt and freshly ground black pepper, to taste

Directions:

Start by seasoning the tofu with salt and pepper in a bowl. Add melted butter and onions to a skillet to sauté for 3 minutes approximately. Toss in tofu and stir cook for 2 minutes. Stir in cheese and cover the skillet for 5 minutes on low heat. Serve fresh and warm.

Nutrition:

Calories 184 - **Total Fat** 12.7 g - **Saturated Fat** 7.3 g

Cholesterol 35 mg - **Sodium** 222 mg - **Total Carbs** 6.3 g

Sugar 2.7 g - **Fiber** 1.6 g - **Protein** 12.2 g

#2 Spinach Rich Ballet

Preparation Time: 5 min - **Cooking Time**: 30 min **Servings**: 4

Ingredients:

- 1 ½ lbs. fresh baby spinach

- 8 tsp. coconut cream

- 14 ounces cauliflower, sliced

- 2 tbsp. unsalted butter, melted

- salt and freshly ground black pepper, to taste

Directions:

Allow your oven to preheat at 360°F/170°C. Start by melting butter in a skillet and toss in spinach to sauté for 3 minutes. Remove the excess liquid and divide the spinach into four ramekins. Divide cream, cauliflower, salt, and black pepper in the ramekins. Bake them for 25 minutes approximately. Serve fresh and warm.

Nutrition:

Calories 188 - **Total Fat** 12.5 g - **Saturated Fat** 4.4 g

Cholesterol 53 mg - **Sodium** 1098 mg - **Total Carbs** 4.9 g

Sugar 0.3 g - **Fiber** 2 g - **Protein** 14.6 g

#3 Pepperoni Egg Omelet

Preparation Time: 5 min - **Cooking Time:** 20 min - **Servings:** 4

Ingredients:

- 15 pepperoni slices

- 6 eggs

- 2 tbsp. butter

- 4 tbsp. coconut cream

- salt and freshly ground black pepper, to taste

Directions:

Start by whisking eggs with pepperoni, cream, salt and black pepper in any bowl. Add ¼ of the butter to a heated nonstick pan. Now pour ¼ of the batter in this melted butter and cook for 2 minutes on each side. Cook more egg pancakes using the same technique. Enjoy warm and fresh.

Nutrition:

Calories: 141 - **Total Fat:** 11.3 g - **Saturated Fat:** 3.8 g

Cholesterol: 181 mg - **Sodium:** 334 mg - **Total Carbs:** 0.6 g

Sugar: 0.5 g - **Fiber:** 0 g - **Protein:** 8.9 g

#4 Nut Porridge

Preparation Time: 10 min - **Cooking Time:** 15 min - **Servings:** 4

Ingredients:

- 1 cup cashew nuts, raw and unsalted

- 1 cup pecan, halved

- 2 tbsp. stevia

- 4 tsp. coconut oil, melted

- 2 cups water

Directions:

Start by finely grinding the cashews and peanuts in a food processor. Stir in stevia, oil and water to make a paste. Add this paste to a saucepan and cook for 5 minutes approximately on high heat with occasional stirring. Dial down the heat and cook on low heat for another 10 minutes. Enjoy fresh and warm.

Nutrition:

Calories: 260 - **Total Fat**: 22.9 g - **Saturated Fat**: 7.3 g

Cholesterol: 0 mg - **Sodium**: 9 mg - **Total Carbs**: 12.7 g

Sugar: 1.8 g - **Fiber**: 1.4 g - **Protein**: 5.6 g

#5 Parsley Soufflé

Preparation Time: 5 min - **Cooking Time:** 6 min - **Servings:** 1

Ingredients:

- 2 eggs

- 1 fresh red chili pepper, chopped

- 2 tbsp. coconut cream

- 1 tbsp. fresh parsley, chopped

- salt, to taste

Directions:

Start by adding all the souffle ingredients to a food processor. Blend until the batter is smooth then pour them into the souffle dishes. Bake them for 6 minutes approximately at 400°F/200°C. Enjoy fresh and warm.

Nutrition:

Calories: 108 - **Total Fat**: 9 g - **Saturated Fat**: 4.3 g

Cholesterol: 180 mg - **Sodium**: 146 mg - **Total Carbs**: 1.1 g

Sugar: 0.5 g - **Fiber**: 0.1 g - **Protein**: 6 g

#6 Bok Choy Samba

Preparation Time: 5 min - **Cooking Time:** 15 min - **Servings:** 3

Ingredients:

- 1 onion sliced

- 4 bok choy, sliced

- 4 tbsp. coconut cream

- salt and freshly ground black pepper, to taste

- ½ cup Parmesan cheese, grated

Directions:

Start by tossing bok choy with salt and black pepper for seasoning. Add oil to any large-sized pan and sauté onion in it for 5 minutes. Stir in bok choy and cream. Stir cook for 6 minutes. Toss in cheese and cover the skillet to cook on low heat for 3 minutes. Enjoy fresh and warm.

Nutrition:

Calories: 112 - **Total Fat:** 4.9 g - **Saturated Fat:** 1.9 g

Cholesterol: 10 mg - **Sodium:** 355 mg - **Total Carbs:** 1.9 g

Sugar: 0.8 g - **Fiber:** 0.4 g - **Protein:** 3 g

Lunch

#7 Pimiento Cheese Meatballs

Preparation Time: 30 min - **Cooking Time:** 20 min - **Servings:** 4

Ingredients:

- ⅓ cup mayonnaise

- ¼ cup pimientos or pickled jalapenos

- 1 tsp. chili or paprika powder

- 1 tbsp. Dijon mustard

- 1 pinch cayenne pepper

- 4 ounces grated cheddar cheese

For the meatballs:

- 1 ½ pounds ground beef

- 1 egg

- 2 tbsp. butter for frying

- salt and pepper

Directions:

In a large bowl, mix all the ingredients for the pimiento cheese. Add egg and some ground beef to the cheese mixture. To combine, you may need to a wooden spoon, or use your hands. We recommend using latex gloves when handling raw meat. Add salt and pepper to taste. Once you used the mixture to form large meatballs, fry them in butter in a pan over medium heat, until they are cooked thoroughly. Use a side dish of your choice (some cooked vegetables would be a great choice), and perhaps serve it with a green salad and homemade mayonnaise. This recipe is for 4 servings and the meal only has 1 gram of carbs (not including the side dish).

Nutrition:

Calories: 660 - **Total Fat**: 53 g - **Saturated Fat**: 0 g

Cholesterol: 0 mg - **Sodium**: 0 mg - **Total Carbs**: 1 g

Sugar: 0 g - **Fiber**: 0 g - **Protein**: 42 g

#8 Baked Salmon with Pesto (Keto Style)

Preparation Time: 30 min - **Cooking Time:** 20 min - **Servings:** 4

Ingredients:

- 4 tbsp. green pesto

- 1 cup mayonnaise

- ½ cup full-fat Greek yogurt

- salt and pepper

for the salmon part:

- 2 pounds salmon

- salt and pepper

Directions:

Salmon is a delicious meal to have, and there are plenty of people who would like to serve it for dinner. Therefore, why not have such a delicious meal cooked in a ketogenic way? The following recipe is for 4 servings and it only has 3 grams of carbs. Sounds interesting? This is a very simple dish - simply cook your salmon how you prefer - in a pan, in the oven, broiler or on the grill. Salmon is best prepared medium-rare - so slightly rare just in the middle. Top it with the green sauce and serve. Enjoy!

Nutrition:

Calories: 182.9 - **Total Fat:** 10.6 g - **Saturated Fat:** 2.1 g

Cholesterol: 48.9 mg - **Sodium:** 247.4 mg - **Total Carbs:** 3.8 g

Sugar: 2.1 g - **Fiber:** 0.6 g - **Protein:** 17.1 g

#9 Camembert Mushrooms

Preparation Time: 8 min - **Cooking Time:** 5 min - **Servings:** 3

Ingredients

- 2 tbsp. butter

- 4 ounces Camembert cheese, diced

- 2 tsp. garlic, minced

- 1-pound button mushrooms, halved

- black pepper to taste

Directions:

Place a skillet over medium-high heat. Add butter and let it melt. Once the butter has melted, add garlic and sauté until translucent, should take 3 minutes. Add mushrooms and cook for 10 minutes. Season with pepper and serve. Enjoy!

Nutrition

Calories: 161 - **Fat**: 13 g - **Carbohydrates**: 3 g - **Protein**: 9 g

#10 Mediterranean Stuffed Chicken

Preparation Time: 35 min - **Cooking Time:** 25 min - **Servings:** 2

Ingredients:

- 2 skinless and boneless chicken breast halves

- ¼ cup crumbled feta cheese

- 2 tbsp. finely chopped roasted red sweet peppers

- 15 ounces roasted bell peppers

- 2 tbsp. thinly sliced green onion

- 2 tbsp. snipped fresh oregano

- ½ tsp. crushed dried oregano

- ½ tsp. ground black pepper

Directions:

In each chicken breast, cut a pocket, usually in the thickest part, then put the chicken breast aside. Take a bowl and mix in it feta cheese, roasted peppers, oregano, and green onion. Stuff the pockets of the chicken breasts with the mixture you now have. Place the chicken breast into a frying pan and let them cook over medium heat. When cooked, the chicken breast will turn white (from pink), and the temperature of the thickest part should be around 170 degrees F. As an alternative, you can use a grill, but the instructions are still the same. Around 15 minutes over medium heat. You will need to flip over the chicken breasts (halfway through) and let them grill for 10 more minutes. Put the chicken aside and let it cool. We recommend veggies as a side dish, but it's really your call if you feel like using rice, or potatoes.

Nutrition:

Calories: 186 - **Total Fat**: 8.6 g - **Saturated Fat**: 2.6 g

Cholesterol: 57.1 mg - **Sodium**: 334.7 mg - **Total Carbs**: 1.5 g

Sugar: 0.9 g - **Fiber**: 0.1 g - **Protein**: 23.4 g

#11 Bacon Frittata with Kale and Potato

Preparation Time: 45 min - **Cooking Time:** 30 min - **Servings:** 6

Ingredients:

- 12 ounces tiny red new potatoes

- low sodium bacon, coarsely chopped

- 2 cups freshly chopped kale

- 1 medium chopped onion

- lightly beaten eggs.

Directions:

In a saucepan, pour some water and add salt and place it over medium heat. Then you will need to add potatoes (peeled and chopped) and cook them for about 10 minutes or until potatoes are tender. After that, make sure you drain them and put them aside. Preheat the broiler. Cook the bacon over medium heat until it gets crisp. You can then add onion and kale and cook them for about 5 minutes. Stir in the cooked potatoes. Take a bowl and crack the eggs into it; add salt and ground black pepper and whisk it until you have a smooth mixture. Place the mixture in the pan and cook it over low heat. When it starts to fry, lift the egg mixture using a spatula around the edges, folding gently. Cook the mixture fully. Place the pan under the broiler (make sure it's about 5 inches from heat). Broil it for around 2 minutes, or until the top side is well-cooked and dried. Next, you will need to preheat the oven at 400 degrees F and let it bake for around 5 minutes. When ready, take the frittata out of the oven and let it cool for about 5 minutes. Serve with fresh fruit or a light salad.

Nutrition:

Calories: 175 - **Total Fat**: 8 g - **Saturated Fat**: 3 g

Cholesterol: 251 mg - **Sodium**: 480 mg - **Total Carbs**: 1.5 g

Sugar: 2 g - **Fiber**: 2 g - **Protein**: 1.3 g

Dinner

#12 Western Pork Chops

Preparation Time: 30 min - **Cooking Time:** 20 min - **Servings:** 4

Ingredients:

- cooking spray as needed
- 4-ounces pork loin chop, boneless and fat rimmed
- 1/3 cup of salsa
- 2 tbsp. of fresh lime juice
- ¼ cup of fresh cilantro, chopped

Directions:

Take a large-sized non-stick skillet and spray it with cooking spray. Heat it up until hot over high heat. Press the chops with your palm to flatten them slightly. Add them to the skillet and cook for 1 minute for each side until they are nicely browned. Lower down the heat to medium-low. Combine the salsa and lime juice. Pour the mix over the chops. Simmer uncovered for about 8 minutes until the chops are perfectly done. If needed, sprinkle some cilantro on top. Serve!

Nutrition:

Calorie: 184 - **Fat:** 4 g - **Carbohydrates:** 4 g - **Protein:** 0.5 g

#13 Stuffed Mushrooms

Preparation Time: 10 min - **Cooking Time:** 30 min - **Servings:** 4

Ingredients

- 4 Portobello mushrooms
- 1 cup crumbled blue cheese
- 2 tsp. extra virgin olive oil
- salt, to taste
- fresh thyme

Directions:

Preheat your oven to 350°F/180°C. Put out the stems from the mushrooms. Chop them into small pieces. Take a bowl and mix stem pieces with thyme, salt, and blue cheese and mix well. Fill up mushroom with the prepared cheese. Top them with some oil. Take a baking sheet and place the mushrooms. Bake for 15 minutes to 20 minutes. Serve warm and enjoy!

Nutrition:

Calorie: 124 - **Fat**: 22.4 g - **Carbohydrates**: 5.4 g - **Protein**: 1.2 g

#14 Garlic Bread Stick

Preparation Time: 10 min - **Cooking Time:** 20 min - **Servings:** 4

Ingredients

- ¼ cup butter softened

- 1 tsp. garlic powder

- 2 cups almond flour

- ½ tbsp. baking powder

- 1 tbsp. Psyllium husk powder

- ¼ tsp. salt

- 3 tbsp. butter, melted

- 1 egg

- ¼ cup boiling water

Directions:

Preheat your oven to 400°F/200°C. Line baking sheet with parchment paper and keep it on the side. Beat butter with garlic powder and keep it on the side. Add almond flour, baking powder, husk, salt in a bowl and mix in butter and egg; mix well. Pour boiling water in the mix and stir until you have a nice dough. Divide the dough into 8 balls and roll into breadsticks. Place on a baking sheet and bake for 15 minutes. Brush each stick with garlic butter and bake for 5 minutes more. Serve and enjoy!

Nutrition:

Calorie: 259 - **Fat:** 24 g - **Carbohydrates:** 5 g - **Protein:** 7 g

#15 Smothered Pork Chops

Preparation Time: 10 min - **Cooking Time:** 30 min - **Servings:** 4

Ingredients:

- 4 pork chops, bone-in
- 2 tbsp. of olive oil
- ¼ cup of vegetable broth
- ½ a pound of Yukon gold potatoes, peeled and chopped
- 1 large onion, sliced
- 2 garlic cloves, minced
- 2 tsp. of rubbed sage
- 1 tsp. of thyme, ground
- salt and pepper as needed

Directions:

Preheat your oven to 350°F/180°C. Take a large-sized skillet and place it over medium heat. Add a tablespoon of oil and allow the oil to heat up. Add pork chops and cook them for 4-5 minutes per side until browned. Transfer chops to a baking dish. Pour broth over the chops. Add remaining oil to the pan and sauté potatoes, onion, garlic for 3-4 minutes. Take a large bowl and add potatoes, garlic, onion, thyme, sage, pepper, and salt. Transfer this mixture to the baking dish (with pork). Bake for 20-30 minutes. Serve and enjoy!

Nutrition:

Calorie: 261 - **Fat**: 10 g - **Carbohydrates**: 1.3 g - **Protein**: 2 g

#16 Spicy Pork Chops

Preparation Time: 10 min - **Cooking Time:** 40 min - **Servings:** 4

Ingredients:

- ¼ cup lime juice
- 4 pork rib chops
- 1 tbsp. coconut oil, melted
- 2 garlic cloves, peeled and minced
- 1 tbsp. chili powder
- 1 tsp. ground cinnamon
- 2 tsp. cumin
- salt and pepper to taste
- ½ tsp. hot pepper sauce
- mango, sliced

Directions:

Take a bowl and mix in lime juice, oil, garlic, cumin, cinnamon, chili powder, salt, pepper, hot pepper sauce. Whisk well. Add pork chops and toss. Keep it on the side and let it refrigerate for 4 hours. Preheat your grill to medium and transfer pork chops to a pre-heated grill. Grill for 7 minutes, flip and cook for 7 minutes more. Divide between serving platters and serve with mango slices. Enjoy!

Nutrition:

Calorie: 200 - **Fat**: 8 g - **Carbohydrates**: 3 g – **Protein**: 26 g

Snacks

#17 Orange and Apricot Bites

Preparation Time: 10 min - **Cooking Time:** 10 min - **Servings:** 4

Ingredients:

- ¾ cup coconut
- ½ cup almond butter
- ½ cup dried apricots
- 1 ½ cups pitted dates
- 1 cup rolled oats
- 1 tsp. vanilla
- 3 tbsp. orange juice
- 1 tbsp. zest of an orange

Directions:

Preheat the oven to 350°F/180°C and line some parchment paper on a baking sheet. Place the oats on the baking sheet and toast them for a few minutes until they are slightly toasted. While your oats are in the oven, take out the food processor and add in the dates. Pulse until smooth. Add the vanilla, orange juice and zest, coconut, almond butter, apricots, and toasted oats to the food processor. Pulse so that the mixture becomes a smooth consistency. Move contents into a bowl. Use your hands to make little balls out of the batter and place them into a resealable container. Allow these to set for at least 15 minutes and then serve.

Nutrition:

Calorie: 117 - **Fat:** 2 g - **Carbohydrates:** 17 g – **Protein:** 3 g

#18 Zucchini Chips

Preparation Time: 35 min - **Cooking Time:** 25 min - **Servings:** 4

Ingredients:

- 1 pound of organic zucchini
- ⅓ cup olive oil
- unrefined sea salt, to taste

Directions:

Trim the ends of zucchini and slice them thinly. Toss the zucchini in a bowl with the olive oil and salt Place the zucchini slices on a microwave-safe plate and cook for 10 minutes uncovered. Check the chips, and then cook for a few more minutes, until crispy. You can also cook these in a toaster oven, under low heat for a longer amount of time, up to an hour. Allow the chips to cool and then serve with a low-carb dip or dressing of your choice. Enjoy!

Nutrition:

Calories: 80 - **Total Fat:** 6 g - **Saturated Fat:** 1.5 g

Cholesterol: 5 mg - **Sodium:** 320 mg - **Total Carbs:** 4 g

Sugar: 3 g - **Fiber:** 1 g - **Protein:** 3 g

#19 Trail Mix

Preparation Time: 10 min - **Cooking Time:** 20 min - **Servings:** 4

Ingredients:

- 2 tbsp. sunflower seeds
- 3 tbsp. dark chocolate chips
- 3 tbsp. dried tart cherries
- 10 pcs. dried apricots
- ½ cup raw almonds

Directions:

To get make your trail mix, add the almonds, sunflower seeds, chocolate chips, cherries, and apricots to a bowl. Toss all these together and then add it to a resealable container. You can store this mix for up to 1 month.

Nutrition:

Calorie: 216 - **Fat:** 15 g - **Carbohydrates:** 18 g – **Protein:** 6 g

#20 Kale Chips

Preparation Time: 10 min - **Cooking Time:** 30 min - **Servings:** 4

Ingredients:

- 1 tsp. salt
- 2 tbsp. lime juice
- 1 pc. zest of a lime
- 1 tsp. Sriracha
- ¼ cup olive oil
- cooking spray
- 1 bag torn kale
- ½ tsp. pepper

Directions:

Preheat the oven to 400°F/200°C. Take out two baking pans and coat them with some cooking spray. In a large bowl, whisk together the black pepper, salt, lime zest and juice, sriracha, and olive oil. Take out the torn kale, add it to the bowl, and then toss until the leaves are coated with the dressing. Spread the kale onto single, even layers on the baking sheet. Bake in the oven for about 10 minutes, or until the kale is crisp. You can take the chips out of the oven and allow them to cool off.

Nutrition:

Calorie: 102 - **Fat:** 1 g - **Carbohydrates:** 5 g – **Protein:** 1 g

#21 Cinnamon Cocoa Popcorn

Preparation Time: 10 min - **Cooking Time:** 20 min - **Servings:** 4

Ingredients:

- 1 tsp. cinnamon
- 1 tbsp. cocoa powder
- cooking spray
- 1 tbsp. sugar
- ½ cup popcorn kernels
- 3 tbsp. coconut oil
- 1 tsp. salt

Directions:

Take out a one-gallon pot and heat up three tbsp. of coconut oil on medium-high. Add popcorn kernels one by one, and then when one of the kernels start to pop, you know that it is hot enough. Add in the rest of the kernels. Cover the pot with the lid and shake the pot vigorously and frequently to make sure that there isn't any burning. When the popcorn is popped, you can move the popcorn to a mixing bowl. First, make sure your hands are clean, then spray your popcorn with some cooking spray. Using your hands, toss the popcorn to mix well. Sprinkle with the salt, sugar, cinnamon, and cocoa powder. Make sure that the popcorn is coated properly before serving.

Nutrition:

Calorie: 188 - **Fat:** 12 g - **Carbohydrates:** 2.4 g – **Protein:** 1 g

Conclusion

You should have the preliminary information you need to get started with making your own snacks and meals to maximize your weight loss potential and limit your carbohydrates and fat store accumulation.

In conclusion, 16/8 intermittent fasting includes eating just during an 8-hour window and fasting for the staying 16 hours. It might bolster weight reduction and improve glucose, mental capacity and life span.

Eat a healthy eating regimen during your eating period and drink sans calorie refreshments like water or unsweetened teas and espresso. It's ideal to converse with your PCP before attempting intermittent fasting, particularly on the off chance that you have any basic health conditions.

Whether you are only overweight or have already reached the point where you are considered obese, excess weight in the body can lead to several adverse health effects that can eventually cause life-threatening conditions to develop. When excess fat accumulates, weight loss becomes a crucial component of improving health and ultimately extending a person's lifespan.

16/8 intermittent fasting is easy to follow the method of losing weight. It takes you on a clear-cut path to not only lose weight but also helps you in burning a lot of fat in the body.

This intermittent fasting technique is specifically designed to provide holistic health benefits and would ensure that you lead a healthy and active life.

This biggest advantage of this intermittent fasting technique is that it is very simple and easy to follow. You can practice it irrespective of the life of work you do. It will be suitable for you if you have a desk job and equally helpful even if your business line requires a lot of traveling.

It would work seamlessly for a stay at home mom and would work wonders for a working woman with hectic work life. With a little bit of dedication and discipline, anyone can make this plan work for himself/herself.

You can also get all the benefits of the process by following the simple steps given in the book. I hope that this book is really able to help you in achieving your health goals.

You can use different strategies, and we focused on one particularly popular option in this book – intermittent fasting. In particular, we looked at how you can use the 16:8 intermittent fasting technique to help you shed excess body fat, while also building lean muscle mass and improving your overall body composition.

In addition to telling you how you can use the 16:8 intermittent fasting technique for weight loss, I also shared some highly effective and delicious meal options that you can use to ensure you can lose weight successfully while following this particular method of intermittent fasting.

From here, you can start to experiment with the meals that you include in your daily diet. There is no one-size-fits-all option when it comes to including a specific meal plan in your intermittent fasting plan. The guidance I provided you with here will help you better realize how you should get started.

Choose one little thing to try, even if it is just a one-hour regular meal adjustment. Try this and see how it is working for you. Concentrate on what IF approaches have in common, rather than getting too into detail. Sometimes you eat and sometimes you do not do it, that almost summarizes it.

Consider what is going on in your lives. Think about how much training you are doing and how intensively you are doing, how well you are resting and recovering, how well IF fits into your daily practice and ordinary personal operations, and what other pressure needs and life provide. Remember IF one of the many types of diet is that function. But it "works" only when it is constant, flexible, and parts of your normal practice, not a duty, and not a permanent trigger of physical and psychological stress.

You need to be keenly conscious of how your body is responding to an ongoing program of fasting. Your body system will determine what you consume, how much time you consume, how much time you practice, how much calories you consume, *etc.* Considering all these variables will guarantee that you are in command of the program of fasting and, eventually, your weight.

As you continue with your intermittent fasting journey and achieve the goals you set in the beginning, you can develop new goals and work toward a greater sense of health and well-being. Once you have achieved your weight loss goals, you can then turn your attention to maintaining your goal weight or something completely different, like getting off medication that you are on, for instance.

References

Azevedo, F. R. de, Ikeoka, D., & Caramelli, B. (2013, March 31). Effects of intermittent fasting on metabolism in men. Retrieved from https://www.sciencedirect.com/science/article/pii/S0104423013000213

Berry, S., Valdes, A., Davies, R., Delahanty, L., Drew, D., Chan, A. T., ... Spector, T. (2019). Predicting Personal Metabolic Responses to Food Using Multi-omics Machine Learning in over 1000 Twins and Singletons from the UK and US: The PREDICT I Study (OR31-01-19). *Current Developments in Nutrition*, *3*(Supplement_1). doi: 10.1093/cdn/nzz037.or31-01-19

Cardiovascular diseases in Western Pacific. (n.d.). Retrieved from https://www.who.int/westernpacific/health-topics/cardiovascular-diseases

Brown, J. (2018, November 28). Is breakfast really the most important meal of the day? *BBC Future.* https://www.bbc.com/future/article/20181126-is-breakfast-good-for-your-health

Cherney, S. W. and K. (2020, March 29). *11 Effects of Sleep Deprivation on Your Body.* Healthline. *https://www.healthline.com/health/sleep-deprivation/effects-on-body#1*

Moro, T., & Tinsley, G. (2016). Effects of eight weeks of time-restricted feeding (16/8) on basal metabolism, maximal strength, body composition, inflammation, and cardiovascular risk factors in resistance-trained males. *Journal of Translational Medicine, 14(1). doi: 10.1186/s12967-016-1044-0*

Young, A. (2020, January 29). Want To Try Intermittent Fasting? This Method Is Science-Backed & Super Approachable. *mbgfood.*

https://www.mindbodygreen.com/articles/16-8-intermittent-fasting-schedule

Carter, S., Clifton, P. M., & Keogh, J. B. (2018). Effect of Intermittent Compared With Continuous Energy Restricted Diet on Glycemic Control in Patients With Type 2 Diabetes. *JAMA Network Open*, *1*(3). doi: 10.1001/jamanetworkopen.2018.0756

Catenacci, V. A., Pan, Z., Ostendorf, D., Brannon, S., Gozansky, W. S., Mattson, M. P., ... Donahoo, W. T. (2016). A randomized pilot study comparing zero-calorie alternate-day fasting to daily caloric restriction in adults with obesity. *Obesity*, *24*(9), 1874–1883. doi: 10.1002/oby.21581

FastStats - Leading Causes of Death. (2017, March 17). Retrieved from https://www.cdc.gov/nchs/fastats/leading-causes-of-death.htm

Fitzgerald, K. C., Vizthum, D., Henry-Barron, B., Schweitzer, A., Cassard, S. D., Kossoff, E., ... Mowry, E. M. (2018). Effect of intermittent vs. daily calorie restriction on changes in weight and patient-reported outcomes in people with multiple sclerosis. *Multiple Sclerosis and Related Disorders*, *23*, 33–39. doi: 10.1016/j.msard.2018.05.002

Fothergill, E., Guo, J., Howard, L., Kerns, J. C., Knuth, N. D., Brychta, R., ... Hall, K. D. (2016). Persistent metabolic adaptation 6 years after "The Biggest Loser" competition. *Obesity*, *24*(8), 1612–1619. doi: 10.1002/oby.21538

Fromentin, C., Tome, D., Nau, F., Flet, L., Luengo, C., Azzout-Marniche, D., ... Gaudichon, C. (2012). Dietary Proteins Contribute Little to Glucose Production, Even Under Optimal Gluconeogenic Conditions in Healthy Humans. *Diabetes*, *62*(5), 1435–1442. doi: 10.2337/db12-1208

Fung, J., & Moore, J. (2016). The complete guide to fasting: heal your body through intermittent, alternate-day, and extended fasting.

Fung, J., Fung, J., & Fung, J. (2019, September 26). Dr. Jason Fung: Does fasting burn muscle? Retrieved from https://www.dietdoctor.com/does-fasting-burn-muscle

Gabel, K., Hoddy, K. K., Haggerty, N., Song, J., Kroeger, C. M., Trepanowski, J. F., ... Varady, K. A. (2018). Effects of 8-hour time restricted feeding on body weight and metabolic disease risk factors in obese adults: A pilot study. *Nutrition and Healthy Aging*, *4*(4), 345–353. doi: 10.3233/nha-170036

Glick, D., Barth, S., & Macleod, K. F. (2010). Autophagy: cellular and molecular mechanisms. *The Journal of Pathology*, *221*(1), 3–12. doi: 10.1002/path.2697

Guo, E. L., & Katta, R. (2017). Diet and hair loss: effects of nutrient deficiency and supplement use. *Dermatology Practical & Conceptual*, 1–10. doi: 10.5826/dpc.0701a01

Habib, G., Badarny, S., Khreish, M., Khazin, F., Shehadeh, V., Hakim, G., & Artul, S. (2014). The Impact of Ramadan Fast on Patients With Gout. *JCR: Journal of Clinical Rheumatology*, *20*(7), 353–356. doi: 10.1097/rhu.0000000000000172

Hair Regrowth & Intermittent Fasting: Could This Help? (2020, January 15). Retrieved from https://www.hshairclinic.co.uk/news/will-intermittent-fasting-really-cause-my-hair-to-regrow/

Hjorth, M. F., Astrup, A., Zohar, Y., Urban, L. E., Sayer, R. D., Patterson, B. W., ... Hill, J. O. (2018). Personalized nutrition: pretreatment glucose metabolism determines individual long-term weight loss responsiveness in individuals with obesity on low-carbohydrate versus low-fat diet. *International Journal of Obesity*, *43*(10), 2037–2044. doi: 10.1038/s41366-018-0298-4

How to Stop Intermittent Fasting Headaches. (2020, January 29). Retrieved from https://dofasting.com/blog/intermittent-fasting-headache/

Huda. (2019, January 19). Do Muslim Children Fast During Ramadan? Retrieved from https://www.learnreligions.com/children-and-fasting-during-ramadan-2004614

Hypoglycaemia. (n.d.). Retrieved from https://www.migrainetrust.org/about-migraine/trigger-factors/hypoglycaemia/

IDF Diabetes Atlas 9th edition 2019. (n.d.). Retrieved from https://www.diabetesatlas.org/

Johnson, J. B., Summer, W., Cutler, R. G., Martin, B., Hyun, D.-H., Dixit, V. D., ... Mattson, M. P. (2007). Alternate day calorie restriction improves clinical findings and reduces markers of oxidative stress and inflammation in overweight adults with moderate asthma. *Free Radical Biology and Medicine*, *42*(5), 665–674. doi: 10.1016/j.freeradbiomed.2006.12.005

Klok, M. D., Jakobsdottir, S., & Drent, M. L. (2007). The role of leptin and ghrelin in the regulation of food intake and body weight in humans: a review. *Obesity Reviews*, *8*(1), 21–34. doi: 10.1111/j.1467-789x.2006.00270.x

Knuth, N. D., Johannsen, D. L., Tamboli, R. A., Marks-Shulman, P. A., Huizenga, R., Chen, K. Y., ... Hall, K. D. (2014). Metabolic adaptation following massive weight loss is related to the degree of energy imbalance and changes in circulating leptin. *Obesity*. doi: 10.1002/oby.20900

Land, S. (2018). Metabolic Autophagy: Practice Intermittent Fasting and Resistance Training to Build Muscle and Promote Longevity. *Independently Published.*

Lanham-New, S. A. (2009). *Introduction to Human Nutrition* (Second). Wiley-Blackwell.

Livingston, G. (2015). Never binge again: reprogram yourself to think like a permanently thin person, stop overeating and binge eating and stick to the food plan of your choice! *North Charleston, SC: CreateSpace Independent Publishing Platform.*

Maltz, M. (1960). Psycho-cybernetic principles: a new way to get more living out of life. *Chatsworth, CA: Wilshire Book Co.*

Mattson, M. P., Longo, V. D., & Harvie, M. (2017). Impact of intermittent fasting on health and disease processes. *Ageing Research Reviews, 39,* 46–58. doi: 10.1016/j.arr.2016.10.005

Nedeltcheva, A. V., Kilkus, J. M., Imperial, J., Schoeller, D. A., & Penev, P. D. (2010). Insufficient Sleep Undermines Dietary Efforts to Reduce Adiposity. *Annals of Internal Medicine, 153*(7), 435. doi: 10.7326/0003-4819-153-7-201010050-00006

Qi, L. (2014). Personalized nutrition and obesity. *Annals of Medicine, 46*(5), 247–252. doi: 10.3109/07853890.2014.891802

Reporter, D. M. (2013, September 16). Diet starts today... and ends on Friday: How we quickly slip back into bad eating habits within a few days. Retrieved from https://www.dailymail.co.uk/news/article-2421737/Diet-starts-today--ends-Friday-How-quickly-slip-bad-eating-habits-days.html

Rossi, C. (2019, February 16). The Reason Intermittent Fasting Is Giving You Bad Breath. Retrieved from https://www.popsugar.com.au/fitness/How-Stop-Bad-Breath-When-Dieting-Fasting-44060243

SHELTON, H. (1978). Science And Fine Art Of Fasting.

Shin, B. K., Kang, S., Kim, D. S., & Park, S. (2018). Intermittent fasting protects against the deterioration of cognitive function, energy metabolism and dyslipidemia in Alzheimer's disease-induced estrogen deficient rats. *Experimental Biology and Medicine*, *243*(4), 334–343. doi: 10.1177/1535370217751610

Tibane, J. (2007). Master Your Thoughts...Transform Your Life: thinking styles and practices to achieve ultimate success. *Struik Inspirational, Tiger Valley.*

The Science. (2020, January 6). Retrieved from https://thefastingmethod.com/the-science/

Tokede, O. A., Onabanjo, T. A., Yansane, A., Gaziano, J. M., & Djoussé, L. (2015). Soya products and serum lipids: a meta-analysis of randomised controlled trials. *British Journal of Nutrition*, *114*(6), 831–843. doi: 10.1017/s0007114515002603

Toro-Martín, J. D., Arsenault, B., Després, J.-P., & Vohl, M.-C. (2017). Precision Nutrition: A Review of Personalized Nutritional Approaches for the Prevention and Management of Metabolic Syndrome. *Nutrients*, *9*(8), 913. doi: 10.3390/nu9080913

Varady, K. A., Bhutani, S., Church, E. C., & Klempel, M. C. (2009). Short-term modified alternate-day fasting: a novel dietary strategy for weight loss and cardioprotection in obese adults. *The American Journal of Clinical Nutrition*, *90*(5), 1138–1143. doi: 10.3945/ajcn.2009.28380

Williams, R.J. (1998). Biochemical Individuality : The Basis for the Genetotrophic Concept. *NTC Contemporary.*

Yu, C. W. and W. (2019, March 8). Gastritis: Causes, Diagnosis, and Treatment. Retrieved from https://www.healthline.com/health/gastritis

Zeevi, D., Korem, T., Zmora, N., Israeli, D., Rothschild, D., Weinberger, A., ... Segal, E. (2015). Personalized Nutrition by Prediction of Glycemic Responses. *Cell*, *163*(5), 1079–1094. doi: 10.1016/j.cell.2015.11.001

Printed in Great Britain
by Amazon

61566522R00078